A MEDICAL HANDBOOK
FOR SENIOR CITIZENS
AND THEIR FAMILIES

A MEDICAL HANDBOOK FOR SENIOR CITIZENS AND THEIR FAMILIES

Howard A. Thornton, M.D.

Auburn House Publishing Company
Dover, Massachusetts

Every reasonable attempt has been made to ensure that the information herein is accurate and timely. Readers are advised, however, to consult their own physician to be sure that the information properly applies to their own particular cases. The author cannot diagnose or prescribe for an individual without actually seeing that person; thus none of the advice herein should be interpreted as a specific recommendation for any particular individual.

Library of Congress Cataloging in Publication Data

Thornton, Howard A.
 A medical handbook for senior citizens.

 Includes index.
 1. Aged—Diseases—Handbooks, manuals, etc.
I. Title.
RC952.55.T49   1988   618.97   87-30821
ISBN 0-86569-171-1 (Paperbound 0-86569-175-4)

Printed in the United States of America

CONTENTS

CHAPTER 4

Stroke   34

CHAPTER 5

High Blood Pressure   39

ACKNOWLEDGMENTS

A debt of gratitude is owed the following individuals, who were generous with their time in reading parts of the manuscript. Their advice and criticism were of great benefit to the author in his work, but the latter is, of course, solely responsible for the content of the book.

Dr. F. Hening Bauer, *obstetrician and gynecologist*
Dr. Melvyn Bert, *ophthalmologist*
Dr. Leonard A. Brant, *urologist*
Dr. Eugene C. Gaenslen, *internist with a special interest in geriatrics*
Dr. Alan H. Greenwood, *dentist*
Dr. Jerome A. Hanowsky, *psychiatrist*
Dr. Philip B. Kivitz, *Director of the Breast Evaluation Center, San Francisco*
Dr. Herbert Konkoff, *urologist*
Dr. William Miller, *ophthalmologist*
Dr. Philip R. Reilly, *Medical Director, Shriver Center, Waltham, Massachusetts*
Dr. Dean Rider, *gastroenterologist*
Dr. Ernest H. Rosenbaum, *Chief of Oncology, French Hospital Medical Center, San Francisco*
Dr. Roger S. Spang, *cardiologist*
Dr. Cynthia Smith, *podiatrist*
Dr. William Talmadge, *orthopedic surgeon*

THE AUTHOR

INTRODUCTION

This book discusses and explains the major health issues that confront senior citizens and their caregivers. It covers the full spectrum of health care—from issues facing those who are physically active on a daily basis to problems of nursing home patients who are bedbound and require total care. Because the practice of medicine has become so complex, presentation of many issues has been simplified for ready understanding by the lay person.

The first of its kind, this handbook ushers in a concept whose time has come: the *active participation* of individuals in their own care. Gone is the age of medicine when doctors were unapproachable purveyors of mysterious nostrums to be accepted without question or feedback. People today are far more educated and sophisticated about health matters—they readily ask their doctor about new medicines or therapies which are presented in the media with increasing frequency.

At the same time, the question is more and more often raised, "Just how much health care is *desirable?*" When the practice of medicine was less advanced, there was frequently little that could be done for an older person with a serious illness. Doctors then could sometimes offer only solace. Now, in contrast, some body parts that have worn out can be replaced and pneumonia can often be prevented with a vaccine. Indeed, it is even possible to prolong life for many far beyond the point where they would wish it. Clearly, it has become important for seniors to understand the nuances of health care, so that they can participate in the decision of how much care they themselves shall receive at any particular time.

This handbook is for people who wish to take more of a role in their health care than has traditionally been the pattern. In this regard, the importance of *preventive* care cannot be overemphasized. During the past decade, especially, we have learned how good diet and health habits can do far more to increase the length and quality of life than modern technology. It is better to exert one's efforts toward preventing disease early, when there is still time to make a difference. For example, age fourteen is when deficiency of calcium intake begins for the average woman. This deficit progresses slowly until menopause, when it begins to advance more rapidly and the ravages of osteoporosis set in. Obviously, it is far better for women to begin the habit of sufficient calcium intake during the teen years than to wait until age 65, when most of the damage—which is irreversible—has been done. (See Chapters 9 and 22, Osteoporosis and Diet, respectively.) For men, the greatest problem in the later years is heart disease—a condition best addressed initially at age 21 by following a diet low in fat and cholesterol. (See Chapters 2 and 22, Heart Disease and Diet, respectively.) In other words, despite the fact that this handbook is entitled *"for senior citizens,"* it can be put to sound use by young adults.

Senior citizens who never had the advantage of good advice on health matters in their younger years cannot turn back the clock. For them, this handbook addresses the areas of potential concern. After age 65, it becomes increasingly important to search for signs of treatable disease. The "complete physical" (Chapter 26) becomes more important, and certain immunizations (Chapter 27) become more valuable. Close attention must be paid to hearing and vision (Chapters 13 and 14), which begin to deteriorate. High blood pressure (Chapter 5) and diabetes (Chapter 11) become more common, and other conditions, such as arthritis (Chapter 10) and constipation (Chapter 12) begin to crop up.

Personal Documentation (Chapter 28), with such items as wallet cards and information bracelets, and Legal Preparation (Chapter 29), with such documents as a Living Will or a Durable Power of Attorney, become particularly important. The Health Survey Questionnaire (Appendix A) represents a distillation of the author's 20 years of experience in treating the elderly. It provides an invaluable database of crucial facts which will enable the treating physician to develop a thorough understanding of a patient's medical profile.

With so many decisions to make, it becomes important for doctors to receive information and guidance from their patients. Would *this* person wish to have tube feedings or be placed in a nursing home? Would *that* one wish the benefit of a flu shot or a pneumonia vaccination? How much help is wanted by those who are overweight, or whose cholesterol is too high? Which of those who smoke really want to quit? Doctors, however, spend much of their time attending to *crisis* situations—heart attacks, broken hips, and the like—and few are able to monitor and coax their patients to have routine exams and to practice preventive care as much as they would like. Consequently, most patients fall far short of benefitting from the full range of medical knowledge now available.

The lesson is clear: Rather than depending passively on one's doctor, it is wise to take an active part in one's health care. Women over 50, for example, need not forego annual mammograms if they are not referred by their doctor. The can *ask* for referral to a screening center (see Chapter 3, Cancer), or go to one on their own (if they do not have a private doctor). Persons over 65 can *ask* their doctor for a flu shot each fall. Persons with a family history of glaucoma especially may want to *ask* their eye doctor for a glaucoma evaluation (see Chapter 26) periodically.

This book can assist both doctors and patients in their mutual efforts to achieve a high standard of health care, not just after 65, but in the years of preparing for that time of life. We recommend that individuals show their primary care doctor this book, in order to further the teamwork approach to health maintenance. We especially encourage everyone to answer the Health Survey Questionnaire (Appendix A) and to present the completed form to his or her doctor.

Chapter 1

WHAT ARE THE ODDS FACING YOU NOW?

Today doctors can use computer programs to predict the chances of your suffering a heart attack or stroke within the new few years. The predictions are based on such facts as your age, blood pressure, and cholesterol level. Programs that take into account additional factors such as your height and weight can provide even better accuracy. Insurance companies, of course, have been doing this sort of thing for many decades, so for a doctor to use a touchtone telephone to obtain a patient's risk profile is not a new concept.

In the broad perspective of things, sending your health data to a computer and getting back statistics running to several decimal places may have some drawbacks. Such "readouts" can give a false sense of security or doom because of the temptation to take the numbers literally. Being told at age 60 that you have a 50 percent chance of having a heart attack within the next 10 years may prompt you to begin preparations to "wrap things up" by age 65. Or, the prospect might bring on a severe depression which could result in a "self-fulfilling prophecy." A far better purpose would be served if similar but more subjective information were used merely to get a general idea of what the future holds. Such a perspective could help all of us to better understand what things are most important for living longer.

Two basic factors determine how long you will live: heredity and environment. If your parents lived to a ripe old age, the chances are that you will, too. And if you have followed good health habits, your chances of growing old likewise increase. With the combination of good genes and good health habits, you are quite likely to live into your 80s or 90s. Upon reaching 65, the average woman can now expect to live about 19 years more, and the average man, another 14 years. Men and women 65 and older suffer from the chronic conditions shown in Exhibit 1–1; the leading causes of death for persons 65 and older are shown in Exhibit 1–2.

The chapters in Part I of this book outline the major conditions which strike senior citizens, beginning with those that are life-threatening. The incidence of heart disease, the number one killer, is greatly increased by high blood pressure, a high cholesterol level, and being overweight. Other major illnesses follow at a considerable distance with cancer, strokes, and lung disease taking a collective "second place." Equally, if not more important than the diseases themselves, are a person's health habits. Smoking,

Exhibit 1–1   Chronic Conditions Suffered by Persons 65 and Over

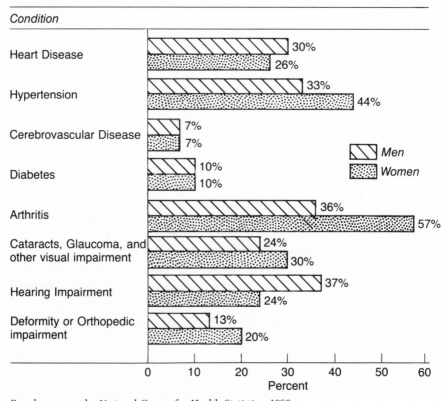

Based on report by National Center for Health Statistics, 1986.

Exhibit 1-2 Leading Causes of Death for Persons 65 and Over

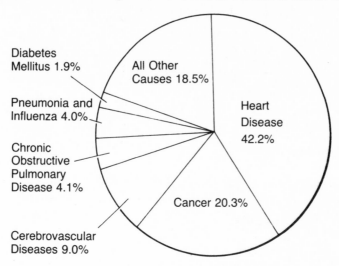

Based on report by National Center for Health Statistics, 1985.

drinking, exercise, and diet are all significant habits that can be more predictive of how long you will live than the genes you inherited. In a large family in which both parents lived to a ripe old age, the sons and daughters who are heavy smokers or drinkers typically die young, while those who shun bad habits tend to live the longest. You might wish to consider your own family tree from such a perspective.

In general, heavy smokers and alcoholics rarely live past 75. Obesity and a poor diet, although less devastating than heavy smoking and drinking, only compound the health problems of persons with such habits. Exercise has a great beneficial effect, but it cannot begin to compensate for the devastating effects of heavy smoking and drinking, and it cannot completely erase the ill effects of obesity and a poor diet. Lack of exercise, however, only worsens matters, regardless of what other factors come into play. One other factor that should not be ignored is stress, which has become suspect—at least in some medical circles—of playing a role no less important than that of cigarettes and alcohol. To summarize, the heavy smokers and heavy drinkers who eat high-cholesterol and fatty foods, who are overweight and exercise little, and who are under great emotional stress are much more likely than their healthy counterparts to suffer a fatal heart attack in their

50s or 60s. If they beat these odds, they are likely to die of cancer, stroke, or chronic lung disease at a later, but still relatively young, age.

Those who have good genes and who follow good health habits are likely to live past 85, but then they are at increased risk for Alzheimer's disease. Although Alzheimer's—known in medical terminology as "presenile dementia"—can strike as early as in the 40s, it increases with age and by 85 afflicts almost one out of four persons. Currently, it is not listed as one of the top 10 causes of death because doctors have only recently begun to recognize it as a distinct entity, and are more likely to sign death certificates with the specific terminal event itself—generally pneumonia—as the cause. Some doctors now rank Alzheimer's as the fourth leading cause of death in adults.

Finally, those few hardy individuals who—besides having good genes and good health habits—are not struck by Alzheimer's, heart attacks, or cancer (being nonsmokers, they do not suffer from chronic obstructive pulmonary disease) often die quietly of a stroke, kidney failure, or some other relatively infrequent cause of death at an advanced age. Sometimes people of advanced age die of "pneumonia," traditionally dubbed "the old man's friend." However, pneumonia as a terminal event—aside from heavy smokers who end up with chronic lung disease—generally occurs only in debilitated individuals for whom some other underlying process, such as cancer, heart failure, Alzheimer's, or plain "old age," has brought about a failure to thrive. Such persons become so weakened that they are unable to clear their lungs of secretions, which stagnate and become infected.

If all this seems a bit depressing to contemplate, one should not lose sight of the ultimate purpose of this book: to survey the major conditions which strike in later life and learn how to avoid them, or at least diminish their impact.

Part I

MEDICAL PROBLEMS: DIAGNOSIS AND TREATMENT

Chapter 2

HEART DISEASE

Heart disease is the leading cause of death in older persons. Each year, about one and a half million adults—most of them over the age of 65—suffer heart attacks. About 36 percent die, and almost half of those who die do so suddenly, without any warning.

What Is a Heart Attack?

A heart attack occurs when there is a sudden loss of blood supply to part of the heart muscle. This event is usually caused by a blood clot in one of the arteries to the heart. Like any muscle, the heart requires blood to bring it nutrients and oxygen. When the blood supply is cut off suddenly, severe chest pain usually follows. Heart attack victims describe the pain as a vise constricting the chest, or a rope being pulled tightly around the chest, or a heavy pressure as if someone were standing on the chest. Marked weakness, shortness of breath, sweating, a very pale look, and sometimes nausea and palpitations often accompany the pain. However, about a quarter of the time few if any of these classic symptoms are present. The person may merely look somewhat pale and not feel entirely normal. Sometimes the pain is located in one or both shoulders, in the left arm, in the neck, or in the jaw. At other times there is no pain, but there may be nausea and perhaps vomiting. In some cases, the person may only become aware of having had a heart attack some years later, when a doctor performs an EKG and finds abnormalities. (This does not imply that an EKG must be abnormal for there to have been a heart attack;

sometimes a heart attack can occur even without any EKG abnormalities.) Although heart attacks sometimes are preceded by bouts of chest pain for days, weeks, or longer, they often come without any warning.

One valuable clue for doctors who are trying to decide if someone is having a heart attack is finding a significant change on the heart tracing from its previous pattern. The problem here is that people who are suspected of having a heart attack often end up at a different hospital from the one they usually go to for their medical care. Or, they may never have actually had a heart tracing taken at their usual hospital, thereby eliminating the possibility of comparing EKGs even if brought there. Often, it is only after a series of blood tests, which may take two or three days, that doctors can conclude with confidence that a heart attack has *not* taken place. Wallet-sized heart tracings that you carry on your person at all times are quite useful to doctors in an emergency when heart attack is suspected. How one gets these is discussed in Chapter 28.

The danger with heart attacks is that they often result in sudden death, due either to weakness of the heart muscle or to heart rhythm disturbances. Although death is sometimes immediate, it may not occur for weeks or more. Deaths most commonly occur outside of a hospital, during the first two hours after a heart attack. For this reason it is important to recognize the signs of a heart attack, and get the person to a hospital as quickly as possible. Many areas now have the "911" system installed, whereby dialing this phone number will put you in immediate contact with the city or county ambulance service. If the person is unconscious and not breathing, the fire department may respond first and perform cardiopulmonary resuscitation until an ambulance arrives.

It is useful for laypersons to learn to perform cardiopulmonary resuscitation (CPR) for just such situations as described above. It may save the life of a loved one. CPR can be learned from your local chapter of the American Red Cross.

Other Manifestations of Heart Disease

In addition to heart attacks, heart disease can manifest itself in several other ways. These are primarily congestive heart failure, angina, and heart rhythm problems. They can come with or without a heart attack.

Congestive Heart Failure

Congestive heart failure is a breakdown in the ability of the heart to pump blood. The weakened heart must beat faster than normal to meet the demands placed on it. Even mild exertion may cause shortness of breath, or the person may experience shortness of breath sleeping flat and need to be propped up on two or more pillows. Leg swelling may occur, and sometimes the person wakes up at night with a feeling of suffocation that eventually goes away after sitting up on the side of the bed. With treatment, most people with congestive heart failure can survive a number of years longer. Without treatment, death may occur much sooner—perhaps in a matter of hours, weeks, or months, depending on the severity of the case. More specifically, even with medical treatment, 62 percent of men and 42 percent of women who develop congestive heart failure die within five years, and 20 percent of such men and 14 percent of such women will die within one year.

Angina Pectoris

"Angina pectoris," also called simply "angina," is caused by lack of sufficient oxygen supply to the heart. It is usually manifested by pain that is similar to the pain experienced during a heart attack, except that the pain is not as severe and is not associated with other symptoms of a heart attack, such as weakness and sweating. The pain of angina typically occurs with exertion or excitement, but not always. It is relieved by rest and by nitroglycerin tablets, which can be placed under the tongue.

Distinguishing anginal or heart attack pain from "gas" pain due to an upset stomach or stomach acid regurgitating up into the esophagus is often difficult. Doctors in emergency rooms sometimes use various medications to calm the stomach or neutralize stomach acid in an effort to make the distinction rapidly.

Heart Rhythm Problems

Persons with heart trouble—especially during heart attacks, but often at other times—may have irregular beating of the heart.

Sometimes the heart may beat too early or too late in sequence; at other times it may beat irregularly in a continuous fashion. Aside from its *regularity* of beating, the heart may sometimes beat too fast or too slow. When the heart beats much below 50 beats per minute, a pacemaker is often implanted to keep the rate higher. When the heart beats much above 100 beats per minute, medication is often administered to slow the rate. Certain kinds of irregular heartbeats or rhythms are particularly dangerous because they can cause the heart to beat ineffectively, so that not enough blood is pumped to vital organs.

Risk Factors for Having a Heart Attack

The heart problems just mentioned tend to be brought on by a number of risk factors, such as high blood pressure, smoking, and too much cholesterol in the diet. The arteries become hard and stiff and clogged with patches of fatty material on their inner walls. These hardened, narrowed arteries are especially susceptible to sudden blockage by blood clots. Although heart attacks are typically caused by a blood clot in one of the arteries of the heart, this is not always the case. Sometimes the artery may undergo a spasm or constriction. Such a narrowing can occur in a completely healthy artery, as well as in one that is already partially clogged. However, persons who already have clogged arteries are at greater risk for a heart attack.

There are two broad categories of "risk factors" for having a heart attack: those that are subject to control, and those that are not. Risk factors over which there is no control are a family history of heart disease, being male, and getting older. Being male is more of a risk under age 60, and especially under age 45. This is because female hormones give women a certain protection against heart attacks during middle age. In later life, however, women become increasingly susceptible to heart attacks.

To a certain extent, other risk factors can be controlled, the most significant being cigarette smoking and high blood pressure. Smoking more than one pack per day doubles the risk of premature death from clogged arteries, with a significant portion of that risk coming from heart attacks. There is a similar increased risk from high blood pressure. These topics are discussed in more detail in Chapter 5 on high blood pressure and in Chapter 23 on smoking.

Cholesterol and Heart Disease

A major factor that contributes to heart attacks is having too much cholesterol circulating in the blood. There are several indicators of too much cholesterol in the blood. One is having a total serum cholesterol level which is too high. Another is having too high a level of the so-called "bad cholesterol"—the LDL serum cholesterol. A third is having too low a level of the so-called "good cholesterol"—the HDL serum cholesterol.

What Is Cholesterol?

To appreciate the importance of the different cholesterol measurements, it is useful to understand a few basic facts about cholesterol. Cholesterol is a special kind of fatty substance that is contained in the membrane of every cell of the body. It is also used in the process of creating sex hormones. Although the body can create all the cholesterol it needs on its own, more than half the adults in the United States end up with too much cholesterol in their blood. This is due in large part to consuming a diet that is too high in cholesterol and fat—especially saturated fat. Excess dietary fat and cholesterol both can lead to elevated blood cholesterol levels. (To learn how to lower dietary fat and cholesterol, see Chapter 22 on diet.)

The excess cholesterol tends to deposit itself on the walls of the arteries, where it causes "hardening of the arteries"—the hard stiff arteries mentioned previously. Since fat and water do not mix, cholesterol, which is a fat, needs to be bound to certain proteins in order to be carried around in the blood (which is mostly water). These special proteins are called *lipoproteins*. Depending on their density, they are called high-density lipoproteins (HDL), low-density lipoproteins (LDL), or very-low-density lipoproteins (VLDL). The proteins of greatest interest in the matter of heart disease are the high- and low-density lipoproteins. Cholesterol bound to the high-density (HDL) lipoproteins is often spoken of as "good" cholesterol, because these lipoproteins *remove* cholesterol deposited on the walls of arteries. The cholesterol bound to the low-density (LDL) lipoproteins is called "bad" cholesterol because these lipoproteins *deposit* cholesterol on the walls of the arteries.

It is known that exercise tends to increase the amount of the "good" (HDL) cholesterol. It is also known that a high fat and cholesterol diet tends to increase the amount of the "bad" (LDL) cholesterol. Although the total cholesterol level is important, it can be misleading if the person has different proportions from the average of the "good" or the "bad" cholesterol. For example, women tend to have higher total cholesterol levels than men, but because of the protective effect of female hormones, they also tend to have less of the "bad" cholesterol.

What to Do About High Cholesterol Levels

Until very recently, many doctors were not convinced that lowering one's cholesterol would do much good. However, research on this subject during the past 15 years or so has amassed overwhelming support for the conclusion that lowering cholesterol levels not only can prevent further "clogging" of one's arteries, but probably can begin to "unclog" arteries as well. Just as the risk of heart attacks rises in an accelerating fashion with higher cholesterol levels, so too does the risk lessen when cholesterol levels are lowered.

When Is Cholesterol "Too High"? Authoritative bodies had constantly argued about which persons should lower their cholesterol, and how they should go about it. Then, in October 1987, the National Heart, Lung, and Blood Institute (NHLBI) published a report for doctors called, "Cholesterol Treatment Recommendations for Adults." Supported by the federal government and 20 authoritative bodies, the NHLBI report provides fairly simple recommendations about classifying blood cholesterol and evaluating patients who are at risk. It also specifies, more clearly than previously, what dietary measures and drug treatments should be taken to lower cholesterol. Unlike earlier recommendations, the treatment approach is the same for adults of both sexes and all ages. However, the report states that there is room for modification based on the doctor's judgment and the patient's preferences, especially for women, young adults (20–29), and persons over 60. Anyone interested in the NHLBI's report or its summary can write for a free copy.*

---

*"National Cholesterol Education Program *Report of the Expert Panel on Detection, Evaluation, and Treatment of High Blood Cholesterol in Adults.*" "Cholesterol Treatment Recommendations for Adults: *Highlights of 1987 Report, National Cholesterol Education Program Adult Treatment Panel,*" October 5, 1987. National Cholesterol Education Program, National Heart, Lung, and Blood Institute, C-200, Bethesda, MD 20892.

Initially, the *total blood cholesterol* level is used to classify all adults. This blood test by itself does *not* need to be performed in the fasting state*—that is, you can have breakfast before you go to the lab. Certain precautions are in order to be sure the test will give the desired information. Only persons following their usual diet and in their usual state of health should be tested. When the blood sample is drawn, they should have been sitting for at least five minutes, and the tourniquet should not be kept in place any longer than is absolutely necessary to obtain the blood. **A level below 200 is desirable, a level between 200 and 239 is borderline high, and a level of 240 or more is definitely high.**

Persons with desirable blood cholesterol levels need only to be educated in a general fashion about diet and risk reduction measures; they are advised to have another blood test in five years. **Persons with cholesterol of at least 200 should have a repeat test within one to eight weeks and the two results averaged.** If a discrepancy is found, a third measurement needs to be made at a later time. Persons with cholesterol levels of at least 240 or those with borderline-high levels (200–239) who are at "high risk" should have a lipoprotein analysis. This requires a 12-hour fast,* except for water and medications.

Who Is at "High Risk"? Persons at "high risk" are those who already have had a heart attack or who have angina or heart rhythm disturbances, or who have at least two other "risk factors." Those other risk factors include:

1. being male;
2. having a family history of premature heart disease (a definite heart attack or sudden death before age 55 in a parent or a brother or sister);
3. smoking more than 10 cigarettes per day;
4. high blood pressure (see Chapter 5);
5. diabetes;
6. severe obesity (being at least 30 percent overweight);
7. a history of definite stroke or other manifestation of clogged arteries somewhere in the body other than in the heart itself; or

---

*Measuring only the total cholesterol itself, or even the so-called "good," high-density-lipoprotein" (HDL) cholesterol, does not require one to be in the fasting state. However, the measurement of triglycerides, or the so-called "bad," low-density-liproprotein" (LDL) cholesterol, *does* require one to have fasted for at least 12 hours.

8. a low HDL-cholesterol level (below 35 as confirmed by a repeat measurement).

If you are a woman and have none of the risk factors 2 through 7, no further testing need be done immediately. However, every man with a cholesterol level of at least 200—even those without risk factors 2 through 7—will need to have a lipoprotein analysis merely to find out if he has a low HDL-cholesterol concentration. (The same goes for a woman with at least one risk factor.) If he does not, and has none of the other risk factors mentioned above, then he (as well as women with "borderline-high" high cholesterol and less than two "risk factors") needs to have his cholesterol measured once a year and begin on the Step-1 Diet that is explained in Chapter 22. Persons who are placed on the Step-1 Diet will need periodic blood tests to measure the body's response to treatment.

Further nuances are involved in classifying persons with border-line or high cholesterol levels. For certain persons, more stringent restrictions than those in the Step-1 Diet may be recommended; some people may eventually be advised to take cholesterol-lowering drugs as well. Although a stricter diet and drugs are not *officially* generally recommended for persons over 60, this is a "grey area" of medicine where more research is needed, and many doctors do not agree with the official recommendations. It is therefore not uncommon for doctors to treat their over-60 patients with drugs if they cannot otherwise bring their cholesterol down.

Certain persons will need to undergo a complete physical and an evaluation to search for special conditions that may be causing the high cholesterol level. Some of these conditions are correctable.

Aspirin for the Prevention of Heart Attacks

Until recently, nothing in the way of medication had been proved to prevent heart attacks in apparently healthy men, although previously, taking aspirin regularly had been found to reduce repeat heart attacks in men who had already suffered their first. However, in January 1988 a large study with American male doctors found **almost a 50 percent reduction in heart attacks in those who took one regular adult-sized aspirin every other day.**

Because aspirin sometimes has serious side effects, it is especially important for persons to consult their doctors before embarking on a program of regular aspirin ingestion. For example, aspirin often causes stomach ulcers and can be dangerous in persons who have bleeding tendencies. However, for those for whom there is no reason not to take aspirin, many doctors now recommend that **men between ages 35 and 70 take aspirin routinely to prevent heart attack. Women who have risk factors for heart attack (such as smoking, high blood pressure, diabetes, a positive family history of heart attacks, or elevated cholesterol) are similarly advised to take aspirin routinely.**

Nevertheless, the reader should be warned that at least one authoritative body—the California Academy of Family Physicians—has concluded that it is premature to expand the findings of the Physician's Health Study to the population as a whole. This is because that study involved a highly select group of male physicians who were at low risk for heart attack, and did not include physicians who were unwilling or ineligible to participate. The reader should also be warned that there was a slight increase in strokes in the doctors in the study who took aspirin, although they still fared much better overall than those who did not take aspirin.

Sexual Problems Following Heart Attacks

Many heart attack victims—particularly men—wrongfully assume that their sex lives are over. The truth is that most heart attack patients need not become "sexual cripples" anymore than they need become "cardiac cripples" confined to wheelchairs. Most of those who are in stable condition and do not suffer from congestive heart failure, heart rhythm disturbances, or unstable angina can with reasonable safety resume a normal sex life about six weeks after a heart attack. Persons, however, who *do* develop symptoms during sexual activity—such as chest pain, or heart palpitations— should stop and rest, and seek medical advice. Persons with stable angina may often benefit by taking a nitroglycerin tablet under the tongue just before sexual activity. A change in coital position to one that is less physically demanding may be recommended for some persons.

Some of the medications prescribed for angina, high blood

pressure, heart rhythm disturbances, fluid reduction, and cholesterol lowering may affect sexual desire or the normal erectile and
ejaculatory functions in men. In certain cases it may be possible to
alleviate such problems by adjusting the dosage or changing the
medication.

Chapter 3

CANCER

Cancer is probably the most neglected area in the health of senior citizens. Unlike high blood pressure, which nearly everyone is concerned about, cancer is a topic that until recently people did not even talk about. Traditionally, and even now sometimes, doctors would not even tell their patients if they had cancer. Unfortunately, because cancer was not talked about it was not thought about either, especially in terms of "could I have it?" As a result, many people did not want to know if they had cancer, and certainly the best way to avoid finding out was never to have a complete checkup.

Cancer is not just one disease; rather, it is many different diseases, all of which have in common the destruction of certain of the body's cells' ability to grow in a controlled fashion. Cancer cells do their damage by growing in a rapid, uncontrolled manner, and often by spreading to other parts of the body. Much progress has been made during this century in medicine's ability to understand, detect, and cure or control many types of cancer—some more than others. However, the aging of the population has done much to counteract this progress, because cancers generally tend to occur in later life and to strike with increasing frequency with advancing age. Overall, deaths from cancer have not changed dramatically. But this is not true with some specific cancers. In recent decades, stomach cancer has become considerably more rare, while lung cancer—primarily due to cigarette smoking—has been increasingly rapidly. Because cancer usually takes about 20 or more years to develop, the recent decline in cigarette smoking is not expected to be reflected in a fall in lung cancer deaths for many years.

Deaths from cancer have been increasing steadily since 1900, and are expected to continue to increase. By the year 2,000, if present trends continue, half a million Americans will die of cancer each year.

Deaths from cancer occur far more often among the elderly. The older you get, the more likely you are to die of cancer. For example, a 70-year-old person is about 100 times more likely to die of cancer than one who is 40 years old. And an 80-year-old person is roughly three times more likely to die of cancer than a 60-year-old. The lesson is clear: if you are over 65, the possibility of having any kind of cancer should be of great concern to you.

Exhibit 3–1 lists the five most common deadly cancers, by age and sex, for persons 55 and older. These cancers, as well as certain others, are discussed more fully in the following sections so that you will have a better idea of the kind of cancer for which you are most at risk.

The Most Common Deadly Cancers

Bowel Cancer

Public awareness of bowel cancer, also called colon cancer, has increased in recent years because of President Reagan's cancer in the right side of the colon—a location where bowel cancer tends to be more "silent." Bowel cancers on the left side of the colon are easier to find because they more often cause symptoms early on.

Exhibit 3–1   Five Most Common Deadly Cancers, by Age and Sex, for Persons 55 and Older

Women 75 and Over	Women 55–74	Men 75 and Over	Men 55–74
1. bowel	1. lung	1. lung	1. lung
2. breast	2. breast	2. prostate	2. bowel
3. lung	3. bowel	3. bowel	3. prostate
4. pancreas	4. ovary	4. pancreas	4. pancreas
5. ovary	5. pancreas	5. bladder	5. stomach

Source: *Vital Statistics of the United States*, 1984.

Examples of such symptoms are constipation and/or diarrhea, or the passing of bright red blood. Cancers on the right side of the colon cause fewer early symptoms because the stool there is less well formed and therefore less likely to cause changes in bowel habits or bleeding from the tumor. Because bowel cancer is the leading cause of death from cancer in women 75 and over, as well as one of the top three causes of death from cancer in both men and women 55 and over, it is especially important for older persons to bring any bowel symptoms to their doctors' attention (see Exhibit 3–2). Unfortunately, bowel cancer will already have spread to other parts of the body in about a third of cases by the time it is found.

Other symptoms of bowel cancer are pain in the abdomen, and weight loss, but these symptoms usually appear only after the cancer has grown quite a bit. Since cancers in the bowel tend to bleed, one way to discover them early is by checking for blood you cannot see. There are several ways to do this, which are discussed in the latter half of this chapter.

Breast Cancer

Breast cancer, the second most common cancer in women 55 and over, is much more common in women after age 40. It is associated

Exhibit 3–2   How the Incidence of Colon Cancer Increases with Age

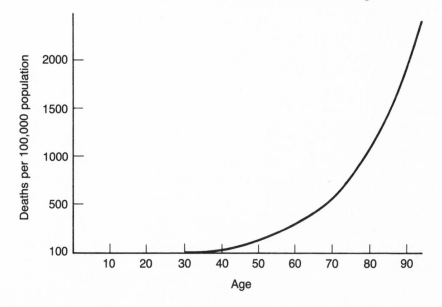

with a family history of breast cancer, with never having had any children, or with having had one's first child after age 31. Seventy-five percent of women probably will never get breast tumors of any sort. Among the other 25 percent who *will* get such tumors, less than a third—7 percent of all women—will get breast cancer. If caught early enough, breast cancer has a very high cure rate. How to find breast cancer at an early stage is discussed in the latter half of this chapter.

Lung Cancer

Lung cancer ranks third as a cause of death from cancer for women age 75 and over. However, it is second for women in the 55–74 age group. Among men 55 and over, lung cancer is the leading cause of death from any particular cancer.

A major problem in the detection of lung cancer is that symptoms usually do not appear until the cancer has become quite advanced, and generally, a cure is not possible by the time it is found. Overall, only 13 percent of those who do get lung cancer live five or more years after it is found. The vast majority of cases of lung cancer are believed to be caused by cigarette smoking. The link between smoking and lung cancer is also discussed in Chapter 23.

Cancer of the Pancreas

Cancer of the pancreas ranks fourth among all deadly cancers for men 55 and over, and for women 75 and over. It is the fifth most deadly cancer for women between 55 and 74. The problem with discovering cancer of the pancreas is that it is hidden deep inside the abdomen. Therefore, it does not generally cause any symptoms until it is too late. Only 4 percent of persons live more than three years after pancreatic cancer is discovered. Smoking is a major factor in getting this type of cancer, with smokers having twice the risk compared to nonsmokers (see Chapter 23). Heavy drinking is also associated with cancer of the pancreas.

Cancer of the Ovary

Cancer of the ovary is the fourth leading cause of death from cancer among women age 55–74, and fifth for women past age 74.

Like cancer of the pancreas, this too is a cancer which is hard to detect early, because it generally gives no warning signs until it is too late. If caught early, 85 percent of women live five years or more. If not caught early, only 22 percent live this long.

Cancer of the Uterus

Cancer of the uterus once ranked fifth as the most deadly cancer for women 55 and over, but it is no longer among the top five deadly cancers for women. A sign of this cancer is spotting in women who are no longer menstruating. There are two types of uterine cancer: cancer of the body of the uterus (the endometrium) and cancer of the cervix (the mouth of the womb).

These cancers tend to grow rapidly. However, they are potentially among the more curable cancers. The key lies in early detection. The five-year survival rate is 66 percent for cancer of the cervix, and 83 percent for cancer of the endometrium. However, for persons who are diagnosed early, the five-year survival rate for cervical cancer is in the range of 80 to 90 percent. For endometrial cancer, the five-year survival rate is 91 to 100 percent—depending on just how early the cancer is found.

Women who have had a complete hysterectomy—that is, removal of the womb and ovaries—do not have to worry about cancer of the cervix, uterus, and ovaries. However, they can still get cancer of the vagina or the vulva, although such occurrences are rare.

Cancer of the Prostate

Cancer of the prostate is the most common cancer among male senior citizens. Estimates are that 90 percent of all men who live to age 90 will end up with this cancer, even if it only lurks silently. The prostate is a male organ about the size of a walnut that is located around part of the urinary passageway. Its rear portion can be felt by a doctor's finger when doing a rectal exam.

Sometimes prostate cancer grows toward the area where the urine passes through the gland, obstructing the passage of the urine. In such cases, the first clue may be an inability to urinate. Or, urination may be very frequent, due to a distended bladder because the urine cannot get out freely. Once the bladder becomes distended, there may be considerable pain in the lower abdomen.

In general, a distended bladder in men is not due to prostate cancer but, rather, to a noncancerous enlargement of the prostate gland. This happens rather commonly in men past the age of 65.

Prostate cancer can spread to the bones. Unfortunately, little is yet known about the cause of prostate cancer.

Cancer of the Stomach

Stomach cancer, the fifth most deadly cancer among men age 55–74, is one reason why it is important to investigate certain ulcers in older men. Sometimes the upper GI x-ray will suggest its presence. The shape of the ulcer is one clue; its location in the stomach is another. When stomach cancer is suspected, a piece of the ulcer is removed and examined under the microscope, a procedure which is done by passing a tube down the throat while the patient is sedated. If the cancer is caught early enough, part of the stomach can be removed and the cancer cured. However, stomach cancer is rarely found early enough for a cure. Stomach pain is one of its first symptoms.

Bladder Cancer

Bladder cancer, the fifth most deadly cancer in men 75 and over, is two and a half times more common in men than in women. Seventy percent of the time there is blood in the urine. Although bladder cancer is difficult to cure, early detection can do a great deal to slow its progress.

Cancer of the Larynx

Less common than all of the above cancers, cancer of the larynx has a very high cure rate if caught early. It is easy to see using a special mirror. Its first symptom is usually hoarseness. In an older person, hoarseness that persists beyond a week or two should be investigated. Persistent hoarseness may sometimes be a sign of thyroid hormone deficiency or benign polyps on the vocal cords.

If they are caught early enough, 95 percent of laryngeal cancers can be cured. In many cases, one or both vocal cords may have to be removed. If both vocal cords are removed, the patient may have to learn "esophageal speech"—produced by trying to speak while belching—and carry a miniature speaker to place over the voice box in order to be heard. But this is a small price to pay to avoid the consequences. If not checked in time, this cancer invades the neck, resulting in a painful and complicated course.

Skin Cancers

Skin cancers are very common. In fact, one-third of all cancers are of the skin. Fortunately, less than one in a thousand of these causes death. The most serious skin cancer is malignant melanoma, a dark mole that turns malignant. If caught early, before it has spread, 89 percent of persons live five years or more. However, once it has spread, only 46 percent live five years or more. Signs to look for are darkening of or an increase in the size of a mole, and especially bleeding of the mole. The only sure way to find out if a mole has turned malignant is to have a biopsy (generally taken by a skin specialist). Often the entire mole, rather than just a piece of it, will be taken off. If it turns out to be a malignant melanoma, the doctor will often go back and remove additional skin around the area and sometimes nearby lymph glands, in case the cancer has already spread. This tumor often travels silently and frequently ends up in the brain, where it may cause a stroke, even years after the original skin tumor was removed.

Because most people have at least a few moles on their body, and many people have dozens or even hundreds of moles, it is not practical for everyone to remove all their moles just to prevent malignant melanoma. Nevertheless, moles do need to be watched carefully, and any changes should be brought to your doctor's attention.

Skin cancers, including malignant melanomas, are becoming much more common. Although a cancer called basal cell is far more common, it kills infrequently. The emphasis here, due to space limitations, is on the *deadly* cancers. From this standpoint, malignant melanoma is the one skin cancer that has truly frightening potential for death.

Early Detection of Cancer

Periodic examinations designed to detect cancer at an early stage are very important because **certain types of cancer have a very high cure rate if caught early, and are deadly if ignored for long.**

Three kinds of cancers are quite common and particularly fit this category. They are breast and cervical (of concern to women only) and colon cancer. We will consider these first; other cancers will be discussed at the end of the chapter. The attempt made here is to fuse the disparate recommendations of various authoritative bodies* with reasonable and practical advice.

An important part of early detection—especially for cancer of the breast, cervix, and colon—is to become aware of cancer's seven warning signals; if you have any of these warning signs, see your doctor:

CANCER'S SEVEN WARNING SIGNALS

1. **Change in bowel or bladder habits.**
2. **A sore that does not heal.**
3. **Unusual bleeding or discharge.**
4. **A thickening or lump in the breasts or elsewhere.**
5. **Indigestion or difficulty in swallowing.**
6. **Obvious change in a wart or mole.**
7. **Nagging cough or hoarseness.**

Breast Cancer

Certain women are at higher risk than others for having breast cancer: all women over age 50; women who have had cancer in one breast (four to five times greater chance of having cancer in the other breast); and women with a history of having had a mother or sister with breast cancer. (It used to be thought that women with fibrocystic problems were at increased risk for breast cancer; now we know that this is not true.) Women who are at higher risk should consult a specialist in breast health care.

All women should take the following precautions: **a monthly breast self-examination; a doctor's exam every two years until age 50, and then once a year after that; a baseline screening mammogram between ages 35 and 39; follow-up screening mammograms every year or two (depending on risk factors) between age 40 and 50; and annual mammograms after age 50.**

---

*The American Cancer Society, the American Heart Association, the American College of Obstetricians and Gynecologists, the American College of Physicians, the American Board of Family Practice, the Canadian Task Force on The Periodic Health Examination, and others.

Breast Self-Examination. Breast self-examination can be taught by your doctor and learned or reinforced from various pamphlets, brochures, and booklets—many of them free of charge (see Chapter 31). Three-fourths of breast cancers are found by women themselves. The importance of doing breast self-examination regularly is to become familiar with what is normal for you. That way, you will be better able to detect any change. It is important to get medical attention for any changes in the breasts—especially a lump or thickening, a nipple discharge, or a puckering of the skin.

The two common methods of examining one's breasts are the circular method (palpating in concentric circles about the nipples) and the quadrant method (dividing each breast into four imaginary quarters, and concentrating on one quadrant at a time). More important than worrying about which method is best is following the guidelines thoroughly and spending enough time. Some anxious women examine their breasts daily or weekly. This is too often, and makes it more difficult to note any changes that might have taken place in the interim.

Doctor's Exam. Regular breast examinations by a knowledgeable health professional increase the chances of finding breast cancer early. However, there is no substitute for monthly breast self-exams, which should also be performed.

Screening Mammograms. Even with the above measures followed in a fastidious manner, breast cancer all too often will have already spread by the time a lump is found. For this reason, x-rays of the breasts—known as mammograms—are important, *in addition* to physical examination of the breasts. The average survival rate for all patients with breast cancer is only 56 percent. However, with the use of mammograms, which are able to detect lumps even before they can be felt, the survival rate increases to at least 97 percent. **No other maneuver or device can find breast cancer as early, as conclusively, as inexpensively, or as harmlessly as a mammogram.**

The two most common concerns about mammograms are the cost and the risk from radiation exposure. The current cost is about $100 to $110 in places that do not specialize in mammograms. However, at screening centers, the cost is about half.

In the 15 years prior to 1987, the radiation dose used for mammograms was reduced 70 times because of better equipment and techniques. Then, in 1987, a new film was developed by

Kodak, which cut the dose still further—by more than half. The current dose is now only 140th of what it was just a little over 15 years ago. Furthermore, the x-rays given during mammograms are aimed at the breasts only, and therefore are not scattered by various organs to the rest of the body, as are chest x-rays. The amount of radiation to the breasts is now miniscule and far below the amount that could significantly increase the risk of getting breast cancer.

You do not need to have a referring doctor to get a mammogram. The radiologists at breast screening centers are licensed to practice medicine in the sphere of breast health and can advise you when and how often to get a mammogram. They can tell you the results themselves if you do not have a private doctor. Breast evaluation centers are rapidly becoming more common—especially in major metropolitan areas. Look in the Yellow Pages under physicians or clinics; or look in the White Pages under "Breast." A typical listing would be "Breast Evaluation Center."

Women who are seen for breast problems such as a lump or breast pain will have the cost of the mammogram covered by Medicare, whereas as *screening* mammograms—where the woman has no complaint—are not currently covered by Medicare.

An Abnormal Mammogram: What Next?   Another concern is what happens after the mammogram is taken and the results are not entirely normal. To get a better idea of what is in store, let us consider more closely what happens when one has a mammogram.

Two views are taken of each breast. One view is vertical, with the x-ray beam passing from head to foot. The other view is horizontal, with the beam passing across the breast. If you go to a breast evaluation center (rather than to a mobile unit), you generally are told the results immediately if the films are entirely normal. If the films are not normal, whether you are told depends on the instructions of the referring doctor. Often the referring doctor wishes to discuss any abnormal results with you in person.

If the results are not entirely normal, the next step depends on the findings. Sometimes the woman has to have additional views taken to clarify a suspicious area. Occasionally, repeat films must be taken because the original ones were technically not very good. This happens only 1 to 2 percent of the time at centers with well-trained personnel, but it can happen up to 10 percent of the time, or even more, in some places. In a breast evaluation center, where the films are developed immediately (as opposed to a mobile unit), any repeat films or additional views can be taken before the woman leaves.

Further studies are usually in the form of additional x-ray films, such as magnification views. Occasionally (most often in younger women), additional studies consist of ultrasound (sound wave) photographs. Sometimes there is a lump which can be felt but the mammogram fails to detect anything; in such cases, to rely on the results of the mammogram as indicating there is no problem can be dangerous. Suspicious lumps need to be investigated, regardless of what the mammogram shows.

It used to be more "the rule" that women with breast cancer would have a "radical mastectomy"—that is, the entire breast, part of the muscle of the chest wall, and all of the lymph glands in the armpit would be removed. Today, radical mastectomies are not as common. Such factors as the size of the lump, its location, and whether it has spread beyond the breast are carefully considered. In some cases only the lump itself will be removed. In other cases, one-fourth of the breast will be removed. Sometimes a course of radiation therapy and/or chemotherapy is given, in addition to the surgery. Radiation therapy is a series of x-ray treatments; chemotherapy is a series of injections. Both treatments are designed to shrink or destroy cancer cells while trying to leave healthy cells unharmed.

The important thing to understand is that having a mammogram does not increase the chances of radical surgery. On the contrary, by catching breast cancer early, a woman is more likely to end up *avoiding* such surgery.

If further information is needed, a fine-needle aspiration for lumps that can be felt may be informative. (This is the removal and microscopic examination of a small amount of tissue and fluid obtained through a thin needle that is inserted into the breast—a procedure that does not necessarily require a surgeon.) Otherwise, a biopsy—a surgical procedure requiring a surgeon—is needed. On the day of the surgery, the woman may have a tiny piece of wire inserted in the breast under x-ray guidance to assist the surgeon in localizing the lump during surgery. The biopsy is often done under local anesthesia, depending on the location.

Cancer of the Cervix

Cancer of the cervix, one of the two types of uterine cancer described earlier in the chapter, is highly curable (almost 100 percent) if caught early. The key to early detection is the Pap smear. **A Pap smear and a pelvic examination should be done annually on all women who have ever been sexually active or who have reached the age of 18. After three consecutive satisfactory normal annual examinations, the Pap test may be performed less frequently, at the physician's discretion.***

One of the main risks associated with the Pap smear is that it will be misread and the woman given false assurance that everything is fine. This problem was recently highlighted in the national press, where it was pointed out that the lack of adequate controls had led to such sloppy reading of Pap smears by technicians that 20 to 40 percent are inaccurate.† Even in the best labs, the error rate is estimated to be as high as 5 to 10 percent, due in part to the fact that Pap smears are notoriously difficult to read. In the meantime, it seems clear that women have only two immediate ways to protect themselves against lab error: Either have their Pap smears done by doctors who use high-quality labs, or be sure to have their Pap smears done with maximum regularity—even in the face of three previous normal annual Pap smears.

Bowel Cancer

Two of cancer's seven warning signals—a change in bowel habits and unusual bleeding—may portend cancer of the colon. However, early bleeding from bowel cancer is so slight that it cannot be seen with the naked eye. For this reason, doctors test stool samples for blood so scant it can only be seen under the microscope. **All men and women should have three tests of stool for microscopic blood once every two years from age 40 to 50, and annually after that.** (Just how stool is tested for blood is discussed on page 30–31.)

What Produces Blood in the Stool? Persons who find out they have microscopic blood in their stool should not automatically conclude they have colon cancer. Only about 27 to 52 percent of such cases test positive for colon cancer, by one reckoning.‡ By

---

*As of March 1988 these are the guidelines of the American Cancer Society, with similar or identical guidelines having been adopted by the National Cancer Institute, the American College of Obstetricians and Gynecologists, the American Medical Association, the American Academy of Family Practice, and the American Medical Women's Association.

†"The Pap Test Misses Much Cervical Cancer Through Labs' Errors," *Wall Street Journal*, November 2, 1987, p. 1.

‡27 percent of cases are persons in their 40s; and 52 percent of cases are persons over 70.

another, only about 12 percent test positive.* Blood can be present in the stool for a variety of reasons. One is improper preparation for the test by eating raw meat (see page 31). Microscopic blood in the stool can also be caused by hemorrhoids, stomach or duodenal ulcers, "nervous stomach," hiatal hernia (a hernia where the esophagus joins the stomach), diverticulosis ("potholes" of the large intestine), and angiodysplasia of the colon (like having tiny varicose veins on the inside of the colon). An important source of bleeding is from polyps in the colon. It is now believed that 90 percent of all colon cancers—if not 100 percent—start with polyps that eventually become cancerous.

Who Is at High Risk? Persons at higher than average risk for colon cancer include those who have already had colon cancer, ulcerative colitis, or colon polyps, or those who have blood relatives who have had these conditions. They need to be examined more carefully and more frequently.

Early Detection of Bowel Cancer. The American Cancer Society (ACS) has very stringent recommendations for detecting bowel cancer in apparently healthy persons. In addition to the annual stool testing for microscopic blood, as just noted, the ACS recommends **an annual rectal exam made by the doctor's finger, beginning at age 40, and sigmoidoscopy (examination of the last part of the colon with a hollow, lighted tube) every three to five years after two annual negatives, starting at age 50.**

The reason other individuals and groups give for not concurring with the ACS is essentially that these additional procedures are "not cost-effective." That is to say, the additional expense and trouble is "not worth it" because nothing will be found in the vast majority of cases. Nevertheless, it seems only fair to present the following facts before dismissing these additional maneuvers as merely "not cost-effective." Colon cancer is the second most prevalent and the second most deadly cancer in America. It is estimated (at the time of this writing) that 41 percent of the Americans who are diagnosed with colon cancer in 1987 will eventually die of it. Yet, according to Dr. Lasalle D. Lefall, Jr.,

---

*This other way of looking at the true percentage takes into account the fact that while about half of the positive blood tests are associated with either cancer (10 percent) or with polyps that may eventually turn cancerous (40 percent), only 5 to 10 percent of the polyps ever do turn cancerous. It should also be mentioned that the procedures by which colon cancer is investigated (sigmoidoscopy, colonoscopy, etc.) are associated with about 3,000 cases of serious illnesses (such as bowel perforation) and 100 deaths annually.

past president of the ACS, only 25 percent of such Americans need die from colon cancer if everyone followed the ACS recommendations, the reason being that the cure rate *doubles* if colon cancer is found before it has spread.

The importance of rectal exams (both finger and sigmoidoscopic) is that colon cancer can be present and still not cause detectable bleeding. Apparently healthy persons who have tested negative for blood in their stools have been screened with sigmoidoscopy and some of them found to have colon cancer.* Just what percentage is controversial depends on many factors. Of course, the older one gets, the greater are one's chances of having colon cancer (see Exhibit 3–2). Sigmoidoscopy, which examines the last 60 cm of the colon, is able to find at least 60 percent of colon polyps and 60 percent of colon cancers.

The reason sigmoidoscopy is recommended every three to five years is that colon polyps take at least five years to turn cancerous. On the average, those that turn cancerous do so over a period of about 10 to 15 years. Those who are concerned about the pain of sigmoidoscopy should be aware that the rigid sigmoidoscopes of the past have now been largely supplanted by the newer, flexible sigmoidoscopes, which cause far less discomfort.

How to Have One's Stool Tested for Microscopic Blood. Those who decide to have their stool tested for blood may be interested to know that a variety of kits are on the market—some quite "civilized" in design. To be the most thorough, testing should be done on stool from at least three separate occasions, and on two separate samples of stool from each of those occasions. This means that you will need to collect the stool yourself on at least two to four occasions, even if one sample is tested by your physician at the time of a rectal exam.

One method requires "fishing out" a portion of the stool with the end of a wooden stick provided and smearing it on a chemically treated card. Another method (HemaWipe) consists of a pad which one uses much like toilet paper. After use, it is folded and sealed. Both these methods require that the card or pad be sent to the doctor. However, there are several self-testing methods where one can see the results immediately in the privacy of one's home. Two—CS-T and E-Z Detect—involve throwing a chemically

---

Western Journal of Medicine, 144 (1986): 756–58.

treated paper into the toilet bowl after the bowel movement. If there is blood in the stool, the paper turns blue. Another—Early Detector—involves spraying specially treated toilet paper, which turns blue if there is blood present.

Three of these kits are available over the counter from your pharmacist (see Exhibit 3–3). Demand for these items is not sufficient for most pharmacies to carry them in stock; so your pharmacist will probably need to place a special order for you. The other three kinds of kits in Exhibit 3–3 must be ordered in quantity from the manufacturer by your doctor.

When testing one's stool for microscopic blood, it is important to follow the directions carefully—especially with respect to diet and medications.* Certain foods and medications have ingredients that can react with the materials in the test to give a false positive reaction or interfere with a proper reaction. One should avoid red meat, vitamin C tablets, aspirin, and iron pills for several days before taking the tests.

Other Cancers

No periodic examinations other than those already mentioned are believed to be so cost-effective that they are recommended by the

Exhibit 3–3 Testing Kits for Microscopic Blood in the Stool

Name of Test	Manufacturer	Type of Test	Availability
Decatest	Fleet Pharmaceuticals	Card and stick	Over the counter
Early Detector	Werner Lambert	Toilet paper and spray	Over the counter
Hemoccult Home Test	Menley & James	Card and stick	Over the counter
CS-T	Helena Labs	Pad for toilet bowl	Doctor must order (800) 231-5663 (800) 392-3126 (Texas)
HemaWipe	Access Medical Systems	Wiping pad	Doctor must order (800) 321-0207
E-Z Detect	NMS Pharmaceuticals	Pad for toilet bowl	Doctor must order (800) 854-3002 (800) 367-4200 (Calif.)

*Except for E-Z Detect, which has no dietary restrictions.

more cost-conscious authorities. However, some other periodic maneuvers are recommended by the American Cancer Society for apparently healthy persons. These include:

- A pelvic examination for women every three years from age 20 to 40; then annually from age 40 upward (to detect cancer of the ovaries—the fourth leading cause of death from cancer among women age 55–74, and fifth past age 74).
- Health counseling and cancer checkups for men and women every three years starting at age 20, and annually from age 40 on (to help detect cancers of the thyroid, testicles, prostate, ovaries, lymph nodes, oral region and skin).
- Taking an endometrial tissue sample from women at menopause if they have been on estrogen therapy or have abnormal bleeding from the uterus or have a history of infertility, failure to ovulate, or obesity.

It has been argued that ovarian cancer is so difficult to detect that even annual pelvic examinations do not significantly increase its detection or improve survival rates. At least, there is no evidence that this is so. In one study, women who had their ovarian cancer discovered as part of an annual screening program nevertheless had very low survival rates. The argument against having annual pelvic exams is that one should not bother just because there is no better way to detect cancer of the ovaries. The other side of that coin is that this examination might be of some value—even if limited—and the *lack* of evidence does not prove there is *no* value to the exam. There is a similar lack of evidence that screening exams for cancer of the oral region, neck, lymph nodes, skin, prostate, and testicles are cost-effective. This is due largely to the fact that these cancers are relatively uncommon. Again, this does not mean that screening exams for these cancers are of no value.

Self-examination for cancers in some of these areas may be an even more valuable way of detecting them early. Testicular self-examination should be done four to six times a year from age 20 through 45. Although there are no specific guidelines for self-examination of lymph nodes, oral region, thyroid, and skin, yearly self-examination would be wise and becomes increasingly important after age 40, since these cancers (unlike testicular cancer) tend to occur more with advancing age. Self-examination for mouth cancer includes looking and feeling for lumps or sores on the floor of the mouth, anywhere on the tongue, the insides of the cheeks, the gums, the roof of the mouth, and the lips. One can use the thumb and index finger to feel the tongue and can look at the inside of the mouth using a mirror. The American Cancer Society offers a variety of educational materials on self-examination free of charge (see Chapter 31).

Even though it may sound like an unnecessary warning, it cannot be overemphasized that it is most important for **women to report any bleeding or spotting from the vagina which occurs after menopause.** Such bleeding is often a sign of endometrial cancer (cancer of the lining of the womb), and about 80 percent of women with this cancer will have abnormal bleeding. However, endometrial cancer is highly curable; with early treatment virtually 100 percent of those who have it can be cured.

Chapter 4

STROKE

Stroke is the third-leading cause of death in the United States after heart disease and cancer. Three-quarters of stroke victims are persons who are at least 65. Indeed, the older you get, the greater your chances are of having a stroke.

"Sudden death"—occurring within a few seconds or a few minutes—does not occur commonly with strokes the way it does with heart attacks. Instead, deaths from stroke tend to occur over a much longer time frame—months to years. The older one is when one has one's first stroke, the more likely that stroke is to be ultimately fatal. For example, among persons under age 65 who have strokes, only 27 percent die within 30 days, and a total of 51 percent die within five years. However, among persons 85 and older who have strokes, 43 percent die within 30 days, and a total of 93 percent die within five years. Strokes are rare before age 55 but become increasingly common after age 65. However, it is not entirely clear whether stroke is an inevitable event which accompanies the aging process. There has been some evidence in recent years—an acceleration in the decline of deaths from strokes—to suggest that this belief may not necessarily hold true. More research needs to be done in this area.

Overall, about half of all persons who survive their first major stroke do not live another five years; 10 percent are likely to have another stroke within one year, and 20 percent within two years. Most people who die following a stroke do so because of heart problems rather than from another stroke. Since many heart problems can be treated, it is important to get proper medical care after a stroke.

Of those who do survive their strokes, roughly one-third are able to return within two years to their usual activities and get about on their own. Most of the improvement after a stroke takes place within the first few months. After that, some improvement continues during the first year or two. Beyond two years, however, any further improvement is unlikely.

What Is a Stroke?

A stroke is the sudden loss of function of some bodily parts because of interference with the flow of blood to brain cells in a particular area. A stroke occurs commonly in older persons when a blood clot forms in an artery in the brain, or in an artery near to and leading to the brain, blocking off the flow of blood in that artery. Or, the interruption in the flow of blood can result from a blood clot that forms elsewhere in the body and travels up to the brain. A stroke can also occur when a blood vessel bursts in the brain, with the resulting collection of blood forming a clot which presses against nearby brain cells, interfering with their normal ability to receive fresh blood.

The most common cause of strokes is high blood pressure. In fact, people with high blood pressure are four times more likely than those with normal blood pressure to have a stroke. Even persons who have only elevated *systolic* pressure are at a substantially increased risk for having a stroke. Other conditions associated with strokes are various kinds of heart trouble; a tendency in family members to have strokes or diabetes; and the tendencies to smoke cigarettes, use alcohol excessively, be inactive, and eat too many foods high in fat or cholesterol.

The likelihood of having a stroke is also associated with the occurrence of a previous stroke or ministroke—what doctors call a **TIA (transient ischemic attack)**. The effects of a ministroke last less than 24 hours. About a third to a half of those who have a ministroke will suffer a major stroke within five years. A large number of these people have a major stroke within the first few months. Many neurologists believe that people who have ministrokes should be hospitalized immediately or studied promptly in order to find out the cause and prevent further damage, such as a severe stroke, which may be fatal.

A full-fledged stroke can be defined as one from which the

person does not fully recover within three weeks. Intermediate between a ministroke and a full-fledged stroke is a stroke that causes loss of abilities for more than 24 hours but less than three weeks. Technically, this is not an actual, full-fledged stroke, just as a ministroke is not. However, many doctors refer to it as a stroke, or a minor stroke, for the sake of convenience.

What Is Affected by a Stroke?

A major stroke always results in the loss of certain mental and/or physical abilities over a relatively short period of time, generally within a few minutes to a few hours. Often, nearby brain cells will begin to take up the functions of those cells that were destroyed, and some degree of recovery may follow afterward.

Precisely what abilities are lost or diminished from a stroke depends on what part of the brain is affected. As mentioned, stroke results from interruption of the blood supply to a part of the brain. When that results from a clogged artery, it is somewhat easier to predict the effect. When the blood supply to the brain is interrupted from a branch of an artery in the *front* of the neck, the result is often paralysis on one side of the body, with perhaps some loss of speech, loss of some vision, and loss of some thinking abilities. There may also be numbness on at least part of one side of the body. When the affected blood supply is from a branch of an artery in the *back* of the neck, many of the same losses may occur, but they typically are not as prominent, although other problems—such as double vision, dizziness, loss of balance, and difficulty swallowing—are likely to result. The ways in which strokes affect people can vary greatly. Some strokes cause only numbness but no weakness; others cause weakness but no numbness. Some strokes cause neither weakness nor numbness but clumsiness of one hand, slurred speech, mild balance difficulties, or drooping of the muscles on one side of the face. Because strokes can cause severe weakness, many stroke patients are plagued by nervousness and depression afterward, and many become socially isolated. A stroke often causes severe economic strain and disruption of family life.

Several common problems afflict stroke patients long after the event. In roughly a quarter of the victims, one hand becomes very swollen and stiff, and the shoulder on that side becomes painful.

This condition usually develops over a period of 3 to 6 months, and eventually goes away by itself, without treatment.

About 5 percent of stroke patients end up with epilepsy, a condition characterized by recurring seizures from abnormal activity in a damaged area of the brain. The first convulsion typically occurs between 6 and 12 months after the stroke. Epilepsy can be controlled with medication.

Preventing Strokes

Strokes can be prevented by considering the risk factors mentioned earlier. Those who smoke should stop. Those whose blood pressure is too high should get it down. Those whose cholesterol is too high should take steps to lower it. Those who are sedentary should exercise more. And those who drink excessively should curb this habit. More detailed advice in these areas is found in the chapters in this book on smoking (Chapter 23), high blood pressure (Chapter 5), diet (Chapter 22), exercise (Chapter 25), and drinking (Chapter 24).

Aspirin to Prevent Recurrent Strokes

Until recently, it was not clear whether persons who had suffered a stroke would benefit from taking aspirin routinely to prevent further strokes. Previous studies had suggested that persons with ministrokes (TIAs) would be at less risk for stroke by taking aspirin regularly. In December 1987 the results from a study in Europe (the European Stroke Prevention Study) showed that daily doses of aspirin and dipyridamole (Persantine) cut the incidence of second strokes by a third. Because previous studies found no benefit from Persantine alone, and because it is a relatively expensive drug, many doctors are reluctant to prescribe it for their stroke patients. Three aspirin were found to be no more effective than one aspirin a day in preventing recurrent strokes. Therefore, most doctors prescribe just one aspirin a day for this purpose.

As in the case of TIAs and previous strokes, it has been found that the taking of a daily aspirin helps prevents further deterioration in elderly patients with multi-infarct dementia (dementia due to a progression of many small strokes which come one at a time, in a stepwise fashion).

Aspirin, of course, can cause stomach ulcers in some persons and can be dangerous in those with bleeding tendencies. It should not be taken routinely except on a doctor's advice. (A related issue—the taking of aspirin routinely to prevent heart attacks—is discussed in Chapter 2.)

Carotid Artery Surgery to Prevent Strokes

As mentioned earlier, strokes are sometimes caused by clogging of arteries in the head, and at other times by clogging of arteries in the neck. When the clogging is in one of the two large arteries in the front of the neck (the carotids), the cause may be correctable with surgery, in which the clogged area is scraped out. However, doctors often disagree over this issue, particularly when it comes to deciding just how much clogging justifies an operation.

Sexual Problems After Strokes

Strokes that affect the dominant hemisphere (the side of the brain opposite one's "handedness") have been shown in some studies to decrease libido. In addition, male stroke patients commonly have problems with libido and potency following a stroke. However, as stroke patients recover and begin to take an interest in resuming a normal life, there is no reason most cannot resume relatively normal sexual functioning. Of course, adjustments may have to be made, in some cases, for inability to assume previous coital positions, because of specific disabilities following a stroke.

Chapter 5

HIGH BLOOD PRESSURE

The blood pressure reading is perhaps the single most important part of the doctor's exam—something doctors check almost every visit. The doctor is generally watching for high blood pressure, a potentially dangerous condition, but one that is perhaps the most easily treatable among all the risk factors for heart and blood vessel problems. Blood pressure is the pressure of the circulating blood against the walls of the arteries through which the blood passes. When the blood pressure is abnormally high, the walls may become damaged or rupture. Several factors can cause blood pressure to rise, including the volume of blood, the condition of the arteries, and the capacity of the heart muscle to pump the blood.

The Harmful Effects of High Blood Pressure

An important reason to control high blood pressure is to prevent stroke. In fact, high blood pressure is the main risk factor for stroke. High blood pressure can also lead to heart attacks, angina pectoris (chest pain caused by inadequate oxygen supply to the heart), and heart failure. The following examples point out the kind of harm high blood pressure can actually do.

Congestive Heart Failure. High blood pressure is the most common cause of congestive heart failure. It places a strain on the heart, causing its walls to thicken or blow up like a balloon. Heart failure sets in when the heart can no longer pump blood out as fast

39

as it comes in. The extra fluid may collect in the lungs, causing shortness of breath, or in the legs, causing swelling there.

Heart Attacks. A heart attack is five times more likely to occur if your blood pressure is high. Although the mechanism linking high blood pressure and heart failure is well understood, just how high blood pressure causes heart attacks is less clear.

Damage to Arteries. When larger arteries stretch from high blood pressure, they become more susceptible to cholesterol deposits, which stiffen and weaken the vessels. In some small arteries, damage comes from thinning or rupture; in others, from thickening. Sufficient thickening may lead to gradual or sudden clogging, especially by blood clots or cholesterol plaques.

Kidney Damage. Narrowing of small arteries may ultimately result in kidney failure.

Damage to the Aorta. The largest artery of the body, which leads directly from the heart, can balloon out from high blood pressure—this is known as an **aneurysm.** Aneurysms can burst with only a few hours' warning—usually sudden, severe pain in the middle of the back.

Eye Damage. Severe, prolonged high blood pressure can damage the tiny blood vessels in the back of the eye, resulting in poor vision.

Damage to Leg Arteries. When the leg arteries thicken and narrow, insufficient blood may reach the feet. When this happens, areas of skin may blacken—known as "gangrene"—typically on the tips of the toes and tops of the feet.

Important Facts About High Blood Pressure

Blood pressure is measured as the height, in millimeters, to which a column of mercury can be lifted. The upper number—the **systolic pressure**—is the *highest* pressure the heart produces as it is contracting. The lower number—the **diastolic pressure**—is the *lowest* blood pressure occurring when the heart muscle is relaxed.

Totally "normal" blood pressure is less than 140/90. For persons 65 to 74, pressure more than 160/95 is considered high. Pressure between is "borderline." A systolic reading of 160 is often considered an upper limit of "acceptable" systolic pressure. There is controversy about what constitutes an acceptable diastolic pressure, ranging from 90 to 100.

About *half* of persons over 65 surveyed have a high blood pressure reading—especially blacks and women. Sixty-six percent of white females age 65 to 74 have high blood pressure of greater than 140/90. The systolic pressure rises 20 points, on the average, between the ages of 60 and 80.

How Important Is Diastolic Blood Pressure?

Historically, doctors have been more concerned with elevation of the *diastolic* blood pressure than with elevation of the *systolic* pressure. It used to be thought that systolic pressure elevation was merely a benign accompaniment of the aging process, and that the damage from high blood pressure was exclusively due to elevation of the diastolic component. Certainly, there is no controversy about the ill effects of elevated diastolic pressures, and the importance of using drugs, if necessary, to treat moderate to severe diastolic elevations. (For definition of "moderate" and "severe" see below.) Whether elevation of the diastolic blood pressure can be considered "more important" than elevation of the systolic pressure is a matter that continues to be debated; much research is needed to settle this issue.

How Important Is Systolic Pressure?

It is now recognized that for persons who have elevation of the *diastolic* pressure, a high *systolic* pressure is even *more* associated with damaging effects. Despite this, only the diastolic blood pressure has been classified by severity:

- **Mild high blood pressure refers to a diastolic reading between 90 and 104.**
- **Moderate high blood pressure refers to a diastolic reading from 105 to 114.**
- **Severe high blood pressure refers to a diastolic reading of 115 or greater.**

When the diastolic pressure rises above 125, doctors become particularly concerned. When the diastolic pressure is normal, there is controversy over whether to treat a high systolic pressure—especially in persons older than 75. Having only the systolic pressure up is thought to be due to hardening of the arteries. Some doctors believe that, even though this may be *common*, it is not *normal*. Therefore, they try to treat high systolic pressure. Others are not so sure. More information will be available in 1992, at the conclusion of a study now in progress.

Can Blood Pressure Get Too Low?

Some people worry about pressures that are "too low." Under ordinary circumstances, blood pressure cannot get too low; pressures around 90/50 are common and generally of no concern. There is one notable exception—a condition called **postural hypotension**. This is a sudden drop in pressure which can occur with a change of body position from lying down to sitting or standing. Older persons taking high blood pressure medications or nerve pills are particularly susceptible to this condition.

Measuring Blood Pressure

The only way to know for sure if you have high blood pressure is to have it measured. Many people assume they "will know" if they have high blood pressure, but most people with high pressure have no symptoms.

It is important that a proper-sized cuff be used when measuring blood pressure. An excessively large cuff will give a false reading that is too low. Those interested in buying their own blood pressure machines may wish to consult the May 1987 issue of *Consumer Reports*, which reviews 36 electrical and mechanical devices.

In older persons, it is important for the blood pressure to be measured both sitting and standing. This is because many older persons—particularly those taking medication—have a significant drop in blood pressure when they stand up. An excessively low standing pressure may cause dizziness or fainting.

Ideally, two or three readings should be taken during an exam and averaged. The pressure should be measured on both arms initially. Sometimes there is a considerable difference between the arms. This may be due to clogging of an artery on one side. In such cases, the higher reading usually represents the true pressure. Except in cases of severe elevation, blood pressure should be recorded on three separate visits before concluding that a person has high blood pressure. To paraphrase the guidelines of the American Board of Family Practice: **a person can be presumed to have high blood pressure if the average of multiple readings taken on at least three separate visits gives a systolic pressure of at least 160 or a diastolic pressure of at least 90.**

To Treat or Not to Treat High Blood Pressure

Elevated blood pressure generally does not need to be treated unless there is a *sustained* elevation. The risk of a heart attack, stroke, or heart failure rises progressively with increasing duration and levels of both systolic and diastolic blood pressure. Treating high blood pressure reduces these events by 90 percent in persons with severe high blood pressure (115 to 129 diastolic) and by 50 percent in persons with moderate high blood pressure (105 to 114 diastolic). In persons with mildly elevated blood pressure, whether treatment with drugs is significantly beneficial, or even harmful, is a controversial issue.

In almost all cases of high blood pressure, the cause is not known. Sometimes there is an inherited factor. In a small percentage of cases, doctors are able to find a cause that can be cured with surgery. The cause in such persons may be a tumor in the adrenal gland, or a problem with the arteries to the kidneys. Otherwise, there is nothing to do except treat the blood pressure itself, or the conditions that make it worse.

There is controversy about when to treat high blood pressure, as well as about when to use drugs for treatment. The greatest controversy is over whether mild and borderline pressure elevations should be treated. In deciding, other health factors, such as smoking, high cholesterol, diabetes, obesity, family history of high blood pressure, a high systolic pressure, or evidence of damage from high blood pressure, such as a thickened heart muscle,* kidney failure,† or visible damage to the retinas must be considered.

---

*Can be inferred from squiggles on the EKG or from a motion picture made by bouncing sound waves off the heart.
†Inferred from a blood test.

If Treatment Is Decided Upon

It is not always necessary to use drugs when treating high blood pressure. In the case of correctable causes—such as excessive smoking and drinking, obesity, too much salt in one's diet, or stress—the pressure may come down by changing one's diet, losing weight, and reducing stress, etc. After perhaps three to six months without success using nondrug methods, it may be clear that medication is needed.

The problem of treating mild pressure elevation with drugs is that "the cure may be worse than the disease." When diuretics, or "water pills," have been used to control mild pressure elevation, one study found 50 percent more people died than those not given *any* drugs—probably due to elevation of blood sugar and cholesterol, and lowering of potassium, which are side effects of such drugs.

In certain older persons, blood pressure cannot be brought down without encountering side effects from the drugs. The American Board of Family Practice states that it is acceptable for certain persons to maintain moderate or even severe levels of pressure in such cases.

The Canadian Recommendations for Treating High Blood Pressure

Although various bodies differ on how to treat high blood pressure, one of the most sensible guidelines is that of a Canadian group,* which differentiates between senior citizens older and younger than 75. For the "younger" group, drugs are recommended if the systolic pressure is 200 or the diastolic pressure is 100. In the "older" group, drug treatment is recommended only if the diastolic pressure is 120. The Canadian group is particularly cautious about treating the "older" group, conceding that little is known, especially regarding high systolic pressure when the diastolic pressure is normal.

Medications for High Blood Pressure

Except in certain complicating conditions such as kidney or heart failure, choosing a drug to lower blood pressure is largely a matter

*The Canadian Hypertensive Society's 1985 Consensus Conference on Hypertension in the Elderly.

of cost, strength of the pill, how often it must be taken, and its side effects. Of course, associated conditions, such as having angina *and* high blood pressure, may be reason to "kill two birds with one stone" by choosing drugs that benefit both problems.

The most common side effects from blood pressure medicines in older persons are dry mouth, drowsiness, and postural hypotension—dizziness and a tendency to pass out when standing up. Postural hypotension, as mentioned earlier, is caused by the blood pressure dropping too low. It is especially likely to happen to a person who, after lying down for a long period, gets up suddenly. It is important, when first getting up in the morning, to sit on the side of the bed for a minute or two before standing up, and then to get up *slowly*. The same is also true at other times of the day.

Sometimes postural hypotension is a signal that one's blood pressure medicine is too strong. If taking too much medicine is the cause, a clue is dizziness that follows shortly after taking the medication—usually within a half hour to an hour. The best way to identify postural hypotension is to have one's pressure taken both lying down and standing. A drop of 15 to 25 points systolic or 10 to 15 points diastolic may be significant.

Blood pressure medications may need to be reduced or stopped during illnesses such as the flu, especially if there is vomiting and diarrhea, and often for a month or two after surgery. It is best, of course, to consult the doctor before stopping any medication. A capsule summary of some of the more widely used blood pressure medications follows.

Reserpine

One major side effect of reserpine is an increase in stomach acid. It also has a tendency to bring on depression in susceptible persons. It can worsen Parkinson's disease (see Chapter 16). In high doses, it may cause nasal stuffiness. Reserpine is useful for treating mild pressure elevations, and it is inexpensive. It is long-acting, taking some two weeks to reach maximum effect; therefore, it is an excellent drug for persons who often forget or refuse to take their medicine every day.

Diuretics

Diuretics, more commonly known as "water pills," are a class of drugs that remove water and salt from the body. The most widely prescribed class of drugs used to treat blood pressure, they are often used in combination with other blood pressure drugs. They are moderate in price. Diuretics are best taken in the morning, because of the need to urinate often for several hours afterward.

Potassium Loss from Diuretics. In the process of removing fluids, "water pills" often remove potassium. Low potassium levels are typically manifested by muscle weakness and leg cramps. Another side effect of low potassium is skipped heartbeats. Occasionally, severe heart rhythm disturbances can occur, especially when the potassium level gets very low. Doctors check potassium levels using a blood test.

Drug Treatment of Low Potassium. To replace lost potassium, supplements are often prescribed. These come in a variety of forms: liquids, powders, effervescing tablets that dissolve in water, coated tablets, and capsules. Many people find potassium in the liquid form nauseating or irritating to the stomach; some even get an upset stomach from the coated tablets or capsules. On rare occasions, coated potassium tablets—particularly some of the earlier preparations—have caused intestinal perforation. The Micro-K brand of potassium capsules seems to be safer in this respect than some older preparations. Even newer, and perhaps more gentle still, is K-Dur, a tablet that dissolves rapidly in the stomach into myriads of tiny time capsules.

Dietary Treatment of Low Potassium. Often, increasing one's intake of potassium-rich foods is sufficient to correct the imbalance that water pills may cause. A list of high-potassium foods is provided in Appendix E.

Alternatives to Potassium Supplements. Persons with sensitive stomachs may benefit from potassium-sparing diuretics. Two drugs of this type are spironolactone and triamterene. Spironolactone may cause enlargement of the breasts, which can be a problem in men. The potassium-sparing diuretics are not as effective as the "regular" diuretics for lowering blood pressure; for this reason they are often combined with them. The potassium-sparing diuretic triamterene and the regular diuretic hydrochlorthiazide are combined in the popular capsule Dyazide. The drug Maxzide has the same ingredients in a different combination.

Other Side Effects of Diuretics. In addition to causing low potassium, water pills tend to make diabetes and gout slightly worse. They also have a tendency to raise total cholesterol levels slightly and to lower slightly the level of "good" (HDL) cholesterol. For this latter reason there has been concern about whether their benefits are outweighed by the increased risk of heart and blood vessel disease. Persons with certain abnormalities on their EKGs have been found to have a higher mortality risk from being on diuretics, even though the diuretics may control their blood pressure.

Methyldopa

Aldomet, the brand name of methyldopa, is a drug that is effective for moderate high blood pressure. It may cause drowsiness that tends to clear with use.

Clonidine

Catapres, the brand name of clonidine, is a drug that acts rapidly— within an hour in certain preparations. It is also available in a sustained-release skin patch, which can be applied once a week. Its most common side effects are drowsiness, dry mouth, constipation, and postural hypotension. It should not be stopped suddenly. It can be taken either once or twice a day, depending on the patient. When taken only once a day, it is best taken at bedtime because of drowsiness.

Hydralazine

Hydralazine is a useful drug for moderate high blood pressure. Its main side effect is a rapid heartbeat. However, this side effect diminishes or is not present in older persons. At high doses, it may cause a reversible syndrome, which includes arthritis and kidney changes. It must be taken at least twice a day.

Beta Blockers

Beta blockers are drugs that lower blood pressure by their concentrated effect on the so-called beta-adrenergic system of the body. This is a select set of nerve fibers which tend to make the heart beat faster and more forcefully. By blocking such nerve impulses, the heart pumps *less* forcefully. This results in lowered blood pressure.

Beta blockers are ideal for certain very nervous persons who have rapid heart rates, because they tend to slow the heart and calm anxiety. They are not safe for persons with asthma, heart failure, or diabetes. Beta blockers are less effective in older than in middle-aged persons. They can bring on depression in susceptible persons. Some drugs in this group tend to cause nightmares. In general, they are more expensive than diuretics. Some are used twice a day; others once a day. They can bring on severe side effects when stopped suddenly. They have a slight tendency to raise cholesterol and triglyceride levels, both undesirable effects. One of the earliest brands of beta blockers is Inderal. Currently, one of the most popular brands is Tenormin.

Prazosin

Minipress, the brand name for prazosin, is an effective drug for mild to moderate high blood pressure. Its most commonly known side effect is fainting after the first dose (postural hypotension), which happens to about one person in 200. This is due to a sudden drop in blood pressure and is generally avoidable if the person is warned to take the first dose at bedtime and stay in bed for an hour and a half. This side effect does not usually recur unless a water pill is taken sometime after the first dose. In such cases, similar precautions must be taken once again. Many doctors are reluctant to use this drug in older persons because of their increased susceptibility to this side effect. Minipress is somewhat expensive and must be taken more than once a day.

ACE Inhibitors

ACE (angiotensin-coverting enzyme) inhibitors, among them captopril, enalapril, and lisinopril, are a more recent and popular class of drugs. Their main advantage over other drugs is their remarkable lack of side effects for most people. The major side effect of these drugs is that in a very small number of persons they may cause kidney failure or certain white-blood-cell-forming problems. However, these side effects have not yet been encountered with the newest drug of this class, lisinopril. Postural hypotension occurs in about one person in 40—most often with the first dose.

These drugs must be used cautiously in older persons, who are more prone to develop this side effect.

Enalapril can be taken only once a day in many cases, especially if taken in combination with a diuretic. Captopril must be taken more than once a day. Lisinopril has the longest half life and needs to be taken only once a day in most cases. These drugs are among the most expensive blood pressure pills. They are excellent for persons who are squeamish about ongoing side effects such as dry mouth and drowsiness.

Calcium Channel Blockers

The calcium channel blockers are most useful for mild to moderate high blood pressure. These drugs block the passage of calcium ions across the walls of certain muscles—most notably heart muscles and the muscles of the arteries. Since the passage of such calcium ions is essential to the process of muscle contraction, one important effect is to dilate the arteries. This causes the blood pressure to drop. Three drugs in this class are nifedipine (brand names include Adalat and Procardia), verapamil (brand name Calan, and others), and diltiazem (brand name Cardizem).

Although these drugs are mostly produced in forms that should be taken three times a day, longer-acting forms, which can be taken only once or twice a day, have become available. Some of these drugs are rather expensive. They are particularly well suited to older persons because they also have certain beneficial effects for angina pectoris and other heart conditions. However, they are not effective for other types of heart problems, such as slowed conduction of impulses. These problems can worsen when drugs of this class are given.

Only verapamil has been approved by the FDA for treating high blood pressure. However, nifedipine and diltiazem may soon become so licensed. Unlike beta blockers, the calcium channel blockers work better in older persons. Nifedipine stands out as the most powerful drug of this class. Indeed, it lowers blood pressure so quickly (two hours) and so much (50 points of systolic pressure, on the average) that is may be *too* strong for many older persons. In younger persons, nifedipine can cause a rapid heartbeat, but older persons do not suffer this effect as much.

Verapamil, and especially diltiazem, have perhaps the least side effects of any drugs used to treat high blood pressure, particularly in patients with healthy hearts. Neither has significant problems of postural hypotension in older persons. Constipation can be a problem, particularly in older persons, and especially with vera-pamil, which has a 15 percent incidence of causing constipation.

Dangers of Abruptly Stopping Certain Drugs

Some medications are especially dangerous if they are stopped suddenly. Clonidine, discussed earlier, is one. Stopping it sud-denly can result in the blood pressure shooting even higher than prior to treatment and in a fast heart rate, headache, palpitations, and perspiration. Similar effects can occur with beta blockers. When such drugs are stopped, they should be tapered gradually, over a period of a week or two. Beta blockers carry the additional danger that in persons with certain conditions, such as migraine headache or angina pectoris, stopping them suddenly can precipi-tate an attack of the condition.

Chapter 6

SENILITY

Senility, also called dementia, is a mental condition of old age in which the mental faculties seem to have regressed back toward infancy. In the strict sense, doctors use the word "senile" to refer to something that occurs naturally with advancing age—such as senile cataracts. But to most people, the word "senile" means the same as demented. And, while many older people become demented, not all do.

Only a few decades ago few people lived past 75. Dementia was not much of a problem, because very few people lived to the point where they might become senile. But today people are living a lot longer. In fact, half the population is expected to live past 75, and half of those are expected to continue past 85. By the year 2000, 17 percent of the population will be at least 65. As a result, senility is already a major problem and rapidly becoming more of one. It is a particularly difficult problem in those families where it strikes, for it affects not just the person who is afflicted, but all the other family members as well.

What has come as a shock to everyone with the aging of our population is how often dementia strikes the elderly. One-fourth to one-fifth of all people over 85 are affected. Some would classify dementia as the fourth major cause of death in senior citizens, after heart disease, cancer, and stroke. In nursing homes, about half of all residents are there because of senility.

Distinguishing Senility from the Normal Aging Process

A variety of normal changes occur with advancing age. These include reduced vision and hearing, less secure balance and endurance, and slowing of the ability to perform physical and mental tasks. Learning new things becomes more difficult and takes longer. But what is learned is remembered, and the size of one's vocabulary remains the same. Furthermore, most older people are still able to go about their business and take care of themselves.

In the cases of senile persons, however, much more than agility, acuity, and flexibility in performing mental and physical tasks is lost. Senile persons become disoriented to time (perhaps thinking it is 50 years earlier than it really is), place (such as thinking they are at home when they are in a hospital), and person (sometimes not even knowing their own name). Their vocabulary progressively lessens, eventually to only a few words, with a few patients losing speech altogether. Judgment is impaired, and the ability to reason is lost. Such persons eventually are unable to manage their own affairs and must be cared for by others. Initially, this involves taking care of business and financial affairs. Then they may need help with more basic tasks, such as shopping, cooking, and house-cleaning. Finally, senile persons often require assistance in dressing, bathing, and even eating.

Although occasionally senile patients are cared for at home in a bedridden state, the intensity of care becomes so heroic that most families place such relatives in a nursing home. The finality of the institutional placement is particularly anguishing in those cases where the person had always pleaded, "Never put me in one of those places—just let me die at home." But when caring for the senile person becomes too much even for "loving" caretakers, it is not easy or even sensible to follow that request. Even the older persons themselves, once faced with the reality that they cannot manage at home any longer, often "change their tune." In addition, the financial realities are that to hire adequate help to care for bedbound persons 24 hours a day at home is two to three times more expensive than nursing home placement.

Alzheimer's Disease

At this point in time, medical science has nothing to offer in the way of a cure for most cases of senility. Indeed, only one-quarter have causes that can be corrected. The major correctable causes are certain vitamin deficiencies and depression, although some would argue that depression is not always curable. The rest are due either to strokes or to a type of senility named after the German doctor Alois Alzheimer, who discovered this particular form in 1906. In fact, half of all senility is entirely of the Alzheimer's type. The one-quarter of incurable dementia that is not entirely Alzheimer's has at least a component due to Alzheimer's. Thus, Alzheimer's disease is the leading cause of senility in older people, and it plays at least some role in 75 percent of all senility.

Diagnosing Alzheimer's Disease

We now know that Alzheimer's disease is an abnormal deterioration of certain nerve cells in the brain associated with the gradual loss of a chemical necessary for normal functioning. As yet, we do not have a "cure" for the disease, although an experimental drug, originally discovered in 1909, has recently been thought to have promise for dramatic improvement in some cases.

Only since about 1960 have we suspected that most senility is caused by Alzheimer's. Part of the difficulty in knowing the precise number of Alzheimer's cases is that we have no real "test" for the disease—at least not in the usual way we think of testing. Rather than being able to draw a blood sample and declare that a person has Alzheimer's, doctors currently can only provide an "educated guess" as to whether a person actually has the disease. The diagnosis is based partly on a battery of tests that may include a CAT scan of the brain. But it is primarily based on a neurological examination of the patient, with a strong emphasis on a history of progressive deterioration. The disease is difficult to detect early but becomes easier to detect as times goes on. A definite laboratory diagnosis—that is, one which is completely objective rather than a clinical impression—cannot yet be made except at autopsy. However, reports are that such a definitive test may soon be available.*

Until recently, researchers believed that the only clues to Alzheimer's were in the functioning of the mind. Thus, tests to determine whether a person might be showing signs of Alzheimer's were based mainly on an interview. The interviewer would look for telltale signs of memory loss that is different from normal "forgetfulness" or other kinds of dementia. Alzheimer's patients

---

*Scientists from The Albert Einstein School of Medicine, at the annual meeting of the Society for Neuroscientists in Washington, in November of 1986, announced the test, which is based on the discovery of an abnormal protein, called A-68, found only in the brains of Alzheimer's patients.

often try to "cover up" for their deteriorating memories, typically replying to questions with "near-miss" answers rather than admitting that they do not know the answer at all. Or, they might blurt out an answer to an earlier question in answer to a later one. More recently, certain physical signs have been linked to Alzheimer's disease. Rigidity of the arms and legs, a tendency to shuffle when walking, taking a very long time in turning, and not swinging the arms as much as normal persons are a few of the physical disabilities that give important clues as to whether a person may have Alzheimer's. Even so, diagnosing Alzheimer's with any degree of certainty early on remains difficult.

Readers should be warned that trying to diagnose Alzheimer's without the expertise of a professional is unwise. Many of the difficulties encountered with Alzheimer's also occur for other reasons. Family members should not jump to a conclusion based on seeing just a few of the above difficulties. For example, forgetfulness and difficulties with words also come with normal aging, as well as depression or anxiety. Difficulties at work can be caused by depression or a medical condition. Difficulties with complex tasks can come about because of depression, a stroke, a brain tumor, or other problems in the part of the brain that handles such functions. Severe depression or stroke can make persons incapable of choosing their own clothing and unable to dress or bathe themselves. Arthritis is another reason older persons may experience difficulties with dressing and bathing. Bladder or bowel incontinence can be due to infection or other problems in these areas (see Chapter 12).

What Are the Chances of Getting Alzheimer's?

Since many nursing home patients who would appear to have Alzheimer's disease never undergo rigorous testing, the number afflicted with the disease is not known precisely. However, one estimate is that about 10 to 12 percent of all persons will get Alzheimer's before they die. There seems to be an inherited factor in some cases; those who have a close relative (such as a parent or brother or sister) with Alzheimer's may have as much as a 50 percent chance of getting it themselves by age 90, according to one study.*

---

*R. C. Mohs et al., "Alzheimer's Disease: Morbid Risk Among First-Degree Relatives Approximates 50% by 90 Years of Age," *Archives of General Psychiatry* 44 (1987):405–08. (For reprints, write to Dr. Richard C. Mohs, Psychiatry Service [116A], Bronx Veterans Administration Medical Center, Bronx, N.Y. 10468.)

What Happens to Alzheimer's Patients?

The course of Alzheimer's has been likened to a child regressing back to infancy. Abilities are lost in the reverse order in which they were gained. Just as an infant progresses from lying to sitting to walking, so do Alzheimer's patients progress—but in the reverse order. A similar reverse progression occurs with memory and speech abilities.

In its earliest stage, Alzheimer's may be indistinguishable from the changes which accompany normal aging—difficulty with remembering dates and names and a general tendency to forgetfulness. As the disease progresses, however, telltale signs begin to appear. Alzheimer's patients are likely to encounter problems going about their daily routine. For example, they may get lost traveling to a new place. Eventually they may get lost traveling to familiar places. Complex matters such as finances become too much to handle. Still later, they may no longer be able to choose their clothing properly or even to dress themselves. Difficulties follow in the areas of bathing and using the toilet. Ultimately, incontinence sets in—first with the urine, then with the bowels. Toward the end, the vocabulary becomes greatly reduced. Sometimes speech is lost altogether, and the person is only able to grunt. In severe cases of Alzheimer's, the person loses the ability to walk and suffers falls which often result in broken hips (see Chapter 8). Seizures may also occur with Alzheimer's, although they can usually be controlled with medications.

In the terminal stage of Alzheimer's, most patients end up in nursing homes. In the final stages they are confined to bed and require total care, including a catheter because of bladder incontinence. They tend to develop stiff muscles, immobile limbs, and bedsores. They may lose weight from eating poorly, since near the end they often cannot swallow. Many cannot even smile.

One of the more disturbing aspects of Alzheimer's disease is the emotional changes which can occur, usually in the later stages. Alzheimer's patients can be tearful one minute and irritable the next. Sometimes they strike a family member whom they love. They may suffer from delusions or hallucinations, and they often become very agitated and unable to sleep.

Making Arrangements in the Early Stages of Alzheimer's

Two important matters should be taken care of early in the course of Alzheimer's disease because they cannot be done later. One is attending to dental needs—such as making a good set of dentures and repairing any decayed teeth—while the person is still able to cooperate with the dentist. Any dental work needed once the patient has become combative will have to be done under general anesthesia. The other concern is making legal preparations for later medical care while the person is still rational. In the early stages, Alzheimer's patients are capable of making decisions about how much medical technology they might like marshaled to prolong their lives. After a certain point, however, the ability to reason is lost. Therefore, while there is time, the durable power of attorney, the legal document of choice for delegating one's health care decisions, should be drawn up. This is discussed in Chapter 29.

The Ethical Dilemmas That Accompany the Terminal Stage of Alzheimer's

When an Alzheimer's patient is terminal, the responsible party is often faced with the ethical dilemma of how much medical care to provide a person for whom there is no hope of a cure, and whose existence may have become ignominious, especially if the person did not make his or her wishes known or legally binding. When death comes, the cause is generally pneumonia or an infection in the urine. The pneumonia is often of the aspiration type, resulting from regurgitating and then being too weak to avoid breathing in ("aspirating") the material into the lungs. Aspiration pneumonia is often easy to diagnose, and usually responds readily to specific antibiotics which can be given in the acute care hospital. Being so readily cured, some patients face repeated hospitalizations for recurrent aspiration pneumonia, rather than dying forthwith from their first bout. The responsible party may therefore have to confront certain ethical dilemmas, which are discussed at greater length in Chapter 29. They include such issues as hospitalization, tube feedings, intravenous fluids, intravenous antibiotics, and cardiopulmonary resuscitation. It is a simple matter to keep a patient comfortable with medication for fever (which can be given by rectal suppository), and with morphine (via a shot, by mouth, or by rectal suppository) for pain or respiratory distress. A major question is whether to withhold food or fluids (which can be given by tube feeding or intravenously, respectively).

Chapter 7

MENTAL PROBLEMS

The material in this chapter attempts to simplify a very complex subject. Therefore, some prefatory remarks are in order. Mental problems are not as "mechanistic" as physical problems. Things are not so simple as giving a drug to slow the heartbeat when it is going too fast. Psychiatric symptoms must be taken in context. The causes can be numerous, and it is difficult to link symptoms per se with treatment by specific drugs. It is important for the patient to have a complete evaluation by a competent professional. One needs to treat the diagnosis more and the symptoms themselves less. This having been said, it is still of some value to discuss the usual treatment of common mental symptoms.

A word of caution is especially needed with respect to giving psychiatric drugs to older persons. The elderly are much variable in their reactions to such drugs, and are much more prone to side effects than are younger persons. Therefore, these drugs need to be given to the elderly in a slow and progressive fashion. With respect to drugs in general, one should pause to consider the fact that in some 30 to 40 percent of cases mental problems in older persons are felt to be *iatrogenic*—that is, caused by drugs which have been prescribed by doctors.

Several basic kinds of mental problems tend to plague older people: anxiety, depression, insomnia, and confusion. These common problems are discussed in this chapter. The chapter also discusses sexual problems of the elderly and loneliness and boredom.

Anxiety

Ordinarily, human beings react to danger with a biological reaction to fight or flee. As part of this reaction, the body moves blood away

57

from the intestines and to the skeletal muscles; the heart pumps faster and breathing becomes quicker. Stress produces similar bodily responses for which we lack adequate outlets. The resulting condition is known as anxiety. Although there are times when it is normal to become anxious, many people let their feelings of anxiety get out of control and become disruptive, to the point where their health is affected. Anxiety disorders, which affect women significantly more than men, become more frequent the older one gets. About 10 to 15 percent of women over 65 have anxiety disorders serious enough to need medical treatment.

Forms of Anxiety

The following emotional disorders are all forms of anxiety.

Phobias. The most common anxiety disorder among women is phobia, or an irrational fear of something; the person recognizes that this fear is irrational. The most common phobia is called **agoraphobia,** or the fear of being in a public place. Women with this phobia are typically afraid to leave home.

Panic Attacks. These are spells that come on suddenly and without explanation. They may include sweating, feelings of choking or not being able to catch one's breath, dizziness, heart palpitations, mild chest pain, and a sensation of impending doom. They generally last a few minutes, but occasionally they last several hours. Sometimes panic attacks may be difficult to distinguish from heart attacks, and require investigation, including hospitalization, to be on the safe side. Doctors use the EKG and certain blood tests as the primary tools to determine if a suspected heart attack has actually occurred.

Generalized Anxiety Disorder. Overall anxiety that lasts more than a month is considered a generalized anxiety disorder. The person may suffer from excessive worries or fears, irritability, difficulty concentrating, and distractibility. Jitteriness, heart palpitations, dizziness, and excessive sweating are common, as are headache, blurred vision, difficulty swallowing, nausea, vomiting, hiccups, bloating, upset stomach, shortness of breath, a dry cough, mild chest pain, dry mouth, neck pain, fatigue, and trouble sleeping.

Treatment of Anxiety Disorders

Anxiety can be treated with drugs, by nondrug means, or a combination of both.

Nondrug Treatments. One way of treating anxiety is through psychotherapy—the guided treatment of a mental disorder by a health professional, using communication as the tool. Some kinds of psychotherapy try to get at the underlying problems which are causing the anxiety. Another nondrug method of treatment is behavior modification therapy. This is commonly used to treat phobias. It involves "desensitization," or getting the person to confront the feared object or situation. Anxiety can be relieved in other ways, such as changing jobs or eliminating the situation which may be causing the anxiety. Exercise may also be of benefit in reducing anxiety.

Drug Treatments. The drug Xanax is useful in the treatment of mild agoraphobia, although it is best used for only short periods, because it can be habit forming. Xanax may also be useful in treating panic disorders. For more severe cases of agoraphobia, Tofranil is helpful. This drug is given at bedtime, and often causes drowsiness. Thus, it may help with associated sleeping difficulties. Nevertheless, its effects last throughout the next day. As with most antidepressant drugs, it takes about three weeks to reach its maximum effect.

Generalized anxiety disorders are best treated by Xanax or Ativan. Ativan especially may have side effects when stopped suddenly, so it should be tapered gradually.

Mellaril is quite useful in treating anxiety in persons with mental confusion because it has a sedating effect and does not increase confusion the way the usual anti-anxiety drugs often do.

Depression

Depression is sometimes difficult to diagnose because depressed patients do not always walk into the doctor's office complaining that they feel depressed. They may merely complain of feeling tired, of having digestion problems and trouble sleeping, and of various aches and pains. The diagnosis is even more difficult when their mood is irritability or anger rather than sadness. Often the doctor may become "sidetracked" trying to deal with bodily aches and pains. Sometimes persons who are thought to be senile are merely depressed. Distinguishing between dementia and severe depression is often difficult; sometimes the diagnosis of depression is made only after antidepressant drugs are given on a trial basis. Diagnosing depression requires considering many problems in several areas at the same time. Estimates are that at least 10 percent of elderly people who live alone suffer from severe depression.

Although it is an exception rather than the rule, occasionally certain drugs bring on depression in susceptible persons. Exhibit 7–1 lists some of the drugs that have been particularly known to contribute to depression.

Minor depressive episodes commonly follow an important change in one's personal life, such as divorce or the death of a loved one. When depression becomes severe enough and lasts long enough, doctors call it a major depressive episode.

The Major Depressive Episode

The American Psychiatric Association defines a **major depressive episode** as a condition in which persons have a sad or irritable mood which is very noticeable and persistent. In addition, the person must have at least four of the following symptoms present almost daily for two weeks:

Exhibit 7–1   **Some Drugs Particularly Known for Having the Potential to Cause Depression in Susceptible Persons**

High blood pressure medications:
  beta blockers (such as Inderal)
  reserpine

All steroids (such as Prednisone, cortisone)

Benzodiazepine tranquilizers:
  Valium
  Librium
  Xanax

Barbiturate tranquilizers:
  Phenobarbital
  Seconal
  Nembutal

- poor appetite or weight loss; or increased appetite or weight gain
- trouble sleeping, or sleeping too much
- agitated or slowed physical activity
- loss of interest in usual activities
- tiredness
- feelings of worthlessness or excessive guilt
- difficulty concentrating
- suicidal ideas

Persons experiencing a major depressive episode typically suffer the most in the morning, have trouble sleeping in the middle of the night or in the early morning hours, have poor appetite and weight loss, and have many physical aches and pains—some quite bothersome. They also tend to experience severe slowing of physical and mental activity, and have feelings of guilt and low self-esteem. They lose interest in everything in life and not uncommonly think of—or even commit—suicide. Although elderly people comprise only 11 or 12 percent of the population, they account for some 17 to 25 percent of suicides. Some have frequent crying spells and suffer from inability to concentrate and poor memory for recent events. Some develop a compulsion to overeat rather than undereat; others, who may have strong anxiety superimposed, are overactive rather than underactive. When these symptoms occur for more than a couple of weeks, they may constitute a major depressive episode that calls for medical intervention.

Treatment of the Major Depressive Episode

The so-called major depressive episode can be treated by drug or nondrug methods, or by a combination of both. Minor depressive episodes are not as devastating, and are beyond the scope of this book. A major depressive episode represents a more profound disturbance that has persisted for at least two weeks. Many such disturbances have persisted for years and have gone unrecognized and untreated because of their subtlety.

Nondrug Treatment. Nondrug treatment of major depressive episodes includes psychotherapy and counseling. Sometimes loneliness and social isolation are contributing factors to major depressive episodes. This can be particularly true in cases of persons who are also afflicted with agoraphobia—the fear of leaving home.

Unfortunately, major depressive episodes often do not respond to methods of nondrug treatment. In such cases, drug treatment may provide help, sometimes with dramatic results.

Drug Treatment. A lot of people see depression—even a major depressive episode—as an exaggerated form of normal grief. They believe that drugs are not necessary and that the person can somehow be coaxed to "snap out of it." However, true depressive states are much more complex than this and often require medical intervention.

There is a great deal of prejudice against using drugs for people who have psychiatric problems. Many people believe that drug therapy just "dopes them up," when psychotherapy or some other non-drug treatment might be a better way of getting at the cause of the problem. While this may be true in other mental conditions, it is less often true for serious depression. Here, the use of effective antidepressant drugs not only can quickly confirm the diagnosis, but also put a rapid end to the damage such patients may inflict on themselves or their families—especially when suicide is a strong possibility. About 70 percent of persons with severe depression respond well to drug therapy.

Persons who are going to be treated with antidepressant drugs are advised to have a glaucoma check (and a prostate exam, if male) beforehand, because of potential side effects of the drug. Besides a complete physical with a blood count, urine analysis and chemistry panel, a thyroid blood test is important, as well as an EKG if there have been any heart problems.

Most drugs used for depression are of a class called tricyclic antidepressants, or a similar class called heterocyclics. Two of the most common drugs used are Elavil and Tofranil. However, there are six or seven related drugs also widely used for depression.

To predict which drug will work best for which patient is not easy. In general, however, Elavil and a drug called Desyrel are preferred for so-called "agitated depression"—a combination of anxiety with depression—in which the person is overactive. Unfortunately, Elavil tends to be overly sedating—especially in the elderly. For so-called "retarded depression"—in which the person is "sad," Tofranil and a drug called Norpramin are better. In depressed persons who have sleeping difficulties caused by nightmares or frequent awakening in the middle of the night, Tofranil is a preferred drug. For those who have more difficulty in falling asleep, Elavil is preferred. Elavil is also the preferred drug when weight loss and poor appetite are the most striking features.

Depending on various other medical disorders which the patient may have (such as heart failure, chronic constipation or diarrhea, peptic ulcer disease, or hypertension), different antidepressant drugs are preferred.*

The most immediate favorable effects of antidepressant drugs are improvement in sleeping problems, which occur within a day or two. Pain, headaches, and intestinal disorders usually subside within the first week. After that, improvement in mood and an increase in energy take place within three weeks with the proper dose. Persons who stop their drugs right away are quite likely to feel worse again after three or four days.

Once an antidepressant is begun, it should be continued for at least six months after recovery has taken place. Once recovery has taken place, it is best to taper the dose slowly to half, and then continue for at least 6 to 12 months longer before stopping. To stop, it should be tapered gradually over a period of one or two months. Some patients require a low dose of antidepressant drugs indefinitely to stay in remission. It is important not to drink any alcoholic beverages while taking antidepressant drugs.

Side Effects of Antidepressant Drugs. The most-encountered side effects of the tricyclic and heterocyclic antidepressants are dry mouth, drowsiness, and excessive fall in blood pressure when standing up. In addition, there may be constipation, urinary retention, mental confusion, problems with recent memory, rapid or slow pulse, heart rhythm disturbances, and dizziness. Paradoxically, antidepressant drugs—especially in the elderly—can sometimes make depression worse. They can also cause or increase mental confusion, and can produce psychotic reactions.

Insomnia

Frequency of Insomnia in Older Persons

Sleeping difficulties are common in older persons. Typically, they do not sleep as well as younger people, wake up more often, and

---

*These are listed in J. W. Richardson III, and E. Richelson, "Antidepressants: A Clinical Update for Medical Practitioners." *Mayo Clinic Proceedings* 59 (1984):334. An excellent adaptation is found on page 21 of the monograph, "Depressive Disorders," published by the American Board of Family Practice, 2d ed., 1985. For information, contact Nicholas J. Pisacano, M.D., Executive Director and Secretary, American Board of Family Practice, 2228 Young Drive, Lexington, KY 40505. ph. (606) 260-5626.

tend to be lighter sleepers. They also tend to nap during the day. Many older persons have genuine difficulty in either falling asleep or staying asleep, and such cases may require a doctor's assistance.

Insomnia is often caused by physical or psychiatric diseases. In some cases, such diseases can be cured, and the insomnia with it. In other cases no underlying cause is apparent, and one is left with the problem of treating the symptom of insomnia itself.

Treatment of Insomnia

Nondrug Treatment. It is often best to first try nondrug means of combating insomnia if it is not part of a major depressive episode. Biofeedback or other stress-reduction techniques may be helpful. **Biofeedback** involves learning consciously to control the body's reactions to stress with the aid of machines that monitor those reactions.

An important step in nondrug treatment of insomnia is to establish a regular cycle of sleeping times. One should go to bed each night and awake each morning at the same hour. It is helpful to avoid taking daytime naps. Daily exercise also tends to relieve insomnia.

Many drugs—especially caffeine and alcohol, and also tranquilizers such as Valium—can cause insomnia. So cutting down or eliminating these drugs altogether might relieve insomnia.

Drug Treatment. Sometimes the judicious, occasional use of sleeping pills is useful in treating insomnia. For very mild and only occasional sleep problems chloral hydrate or Benadryl may be helpful. Benadryl is available over the counter in the 25 mg size. For more serious sleeping problems there are much better drugs. The best ones belong to the class known as benzodiazepines. Two benzodiazepines that have short half lives—that is, short intervals at which half the drug is eliminated from, or detoxified by, the body—have recently been developed: Restoril (temazepam), with a half-life of 8 to 12 hours, and Halcion (triazolam), with a half-life of only 3 to 4 hours. The advantage of a short half-life is less likelihood of drowsiness the morning after. The main problem with the above two drugs is that their effectiveness may lessen considerably with time. For this reason, another benzodiazepine with a longer half-life—Dalmane (flurazepam)—is also much in use. Its main side effect is morning or daytime drowsiness. This side effect is less with the smaller, 15-mg-size strength. (It also comes in 30-

mg strength.) Unfortunately, even with this drug, there is loss of effectiveness after several months.

In persons who have persistent sleep problems, the most common complaint is difficulty in *falling* asleep. For such persons, Halcion and Dalmane are better, because they are both absorbed rapidly. In contrast, Restoril is absorbed slowly, and therefore not as good a drug for such persons. It takes two to three hours to reach its peak blood level. Dalmane is the most favored drug for persons with more severe psychiatric difficulties because it maintains its effectiveness better when given regularly over a long period.

It is best to take sleeping pills only every third night. That way, one can determine frequently whether it is necessary to continue their use, and taking them will be less likely to become a habit. It is best to stop using sleeping pills after a few months.

Confusion

Elderly persons cause special problems for their caregivers when they become confused or paranoid, or begin to wander. Confused persons sometimes lose track of the distinction between day and night, and then may wake up late at night and wander about or go for walks. When they leave the house or institution, they often get lost.

Causes of Confusion

Confusion from Memory Deterioration   Many older persons suffer from severe memory deterioration, and lose track of time and even where they are. They also lose the ability to think clearly and learn. Their attention span may become short.

The most common causes of confusion in older persons are Alzheimer's disease and multiple small strokes, called "multi-infarct dementia." A cause of *seeming* mental confusion is severe depression, although the correct diagnosis is often elusive in such persons. Severely depressed persons are often mistakenly thought to be demented.

Confusion from Psychotic and Paranoid States   Many older people develop various degrees of paranoia, ranging from mild suspiciousness to grandiose delusional systems. They may think someone is stealing their money or plotting against them. Others suffer from hallucinations and delusions. Paranoid symptoms by themselves are not a diagnosis, for paranoia can occur with various types of mental disorders.

Treatment of Confusion

Confused persons who are also psychotic—that is, who suffer from hallucinations, delusions or paranoid ideas—often improve if medications are given for their psychotic symptoms. Although an attempt at diagnosing the underlying disorder should be made, the symptoms of paranoia or hallucinations often respond to the drugs Haldol or Mellaril. Mellaril is also the best treatment for confused persons who wander. It should be given in such cases in the late afternoon or early evening, the times after which wandering especially tends to become a problem.

Aside from sedation, drugs such as Haldol and Mellaril may, with prolonged use, cause a phenomenon known as **tardive dyskinesia.** This is a muscular disorder characterized by uncontrollable facial and mouth movements. It often begins with movements of the tongue inside the closed mouth, and therefore can be detected in its early stages by opening the mouth and observing. Tardive dyskinesia generally takes many months of drug use before it begins to appear. Many different drugs can cause this kind of side effect. It is usually reversible with enough time, but not always.

Antipsychotic drugs also can cause **postural hypotension,** a sudden drop in blood pressure when a person who has been lying down or sitting gets up suddenly. Mellaril is particularly known for this side effect.

A new drug claiming to afford some improvement in the mental state of Alzheimer's patients—THA—began a national trial in late 1986 but was halted when some signs of mild liver damage showed up. Subsequently (in January 1988), the Warner-Lambert Company announced that it and the Food and Drug Administration decided to re-start the study, using a lower dose, which hopefully will not cause any liver damage.

Sexual Problems of the Elderly

Although about half the cases of impotence in older men are caused by diabetes, anxiety and depression are responsible for most of the rest. It is important for couples to realize that all men are impotent at times because of such factors as illness, fatigue, or worry, but this should not become a basis for continued fear of impotence, which can become a self-fulfilling prophecy.

It is a myth that interest in sex dies in later life. Studies have shown that more than three-quarters of men and more than half of women age 60–65 remain actively interested in sex. Even among the very old—78 and over—more than half of men and about a quarter of women remain actively interested in sex. Age alone should not be a barrier to sexual expression in the later years.

Loneliness and Boredom in the Elderly

Numerous studies have shown that loneliness and retirement are strongly associated with death in the elderly. Widowed men were found to have a 40 percent higher death rate the first six months following the death of their spouse. Another study found a 70 percent lower death rate among widowed men under 55 who remarried, compared with widowed men who never remarried. The first two years following the death of a spouse are considered the most hazardous in the health of the surviving mate. Among men who retired, a 1980 study found an excess risk of death from heart attacks to be almost double that of men who did not retire.

The importance of religion—both organized and informal—to the health of older persons cannot be overemphasized. One-third to one-half of older persons interviewed volunteered that religion was instrumental as a source of strength in "keeping them on an even keel" when coping with stressful life events. There is a strong correlation between well-being and religious activities and attitudes in older persons—especially those over 75.

In summary, mental problems occur more often in older persons than many realize. It is important to be aware of this fact, and also what kind of mental problems are most common in this age group. Having a "high index of suspicion" for mental disorders in older persons can avoid the trap of concluding that something physical is wrong, when the problem is really mental. For example, persons with panic disorders often have symptoms similar to those of a heart attack; and persons who are depressed are often mistakenly thought to be senile. The root of the problem may lie in social isolation and boredom. Staying involved in the community may be "just what the doctor ordered." Religious activities, both informal and organized, may do much to prolong life and well-being.

Chapter 8

FRACTURES, FALLS, AND MOBILITY PROBLEMS

The term "fracture" is a medical word which simply means "broken bone." In people over 65, broken bones happen mainly to women. Elderly women are *eight times* more likely to suffer from broken bones than elderly men. This discrepancy exists because women are plagued, much more than men, by **osteoporosis,** or thinning of the bones. The bones become brittle, making them susceptible to breakage with only the least bit of stress—sometimes as little as coughing, which may cause broken ribs or broken backbones, or stepping down from a curb, which may cause broken hips. Elderly women suffer from osteoporosis much more than elderly men for two reasons. Women have about 30 percent less bone to begin with when they reach the menopause, and, once past the menopause, they lose bone much faster than men.

The Seriousness of Fractures in Elderly Persons

Elderly persons most often break the wrists, followed by the spine, followed by the hips. Less common are broken ribs and other bones. To a large extent, how old one is determines which bones are most likely to be broken. Wrist fractures have their peak occurrence in the 60s; fractures of the spine in the 70s; and hip fractures in the 80s. However, wrist fractures still remain the most common type of fracture, even at age 80.

By age 65, about 8.5 percent of women still living will have broken at least a wrist, spine, or hipbone. By the age of 80, the figure is one out of four. The rate of hip fractures roughly doubles each decade of life after age 50. After age 80, 5 percent of women suffer hip fractures each year. By the age of 90, a third of women and a sixth of men will have broken a hip.

Some 12 to 20 percent of older persons who break a hip die from complications. Persons who die within one year after a hip fracture are about two and a half times more likely to do so if they are senile. Of those who survive, about half never return to independent living and generally are placed in nursing homes.

The Major Causes of Broken Bones in the Elderly

Broken bones in older persons are primarily caused by the combination of osteoporosis and falls. In women over 50, 80 percent of all fractures are due to osteoporosis. The prevention of osteoporosis is discussed in Chapter 9.

Often, a fall by an older person is dismissed as being of no consequence as long as nothing is broken. However, the fact of merely having fallen is sometimes itself a sign that something is seriously wrong. The fall may be have been caused by a silent heart problem, pneumonia, or a raging urinary infection. Or, it may indicate a problem that could result in recurrent falls. Even if nothing was broken during the initial fall, that is no guarantee the person will not break something in a subsequent fall. Very often, falls in older persons result in broken hips. In fact, 90 percent of hip fractures result from a fall. Injuries, by one accounting, are the fifth leading cause of death in persons over 65, and falls are responsible for two-thirds of these injuries. Therefore, it is important for older persons who have fallen to have a thorough evaluation as to just why they fell.

Aside from falls which have already happened, one should be sensitive to potential mobility problems in the elderly by taking certain precautions to prevent falls from happening. After all, hip fractures often occur with an older person's first fall. In fact, falling down is the most common reason for older persons having to go to the hospital.

Falls with Loss of Consciousness

An important thing for doctors to know, when older persons fall, is whether they lost consciousness at the time. In general, falls in which a person passes out are more serious than other falls. Likewise, it is convenient to classify the causes of passing out as more or less serious, although few causes of passing out are not serious.

The Most Serious Causes of Passing Out

Often, the reason a person passes out is quite serious. Some 15 percent of heart attacks are "silent"—without any pain. The only indication of the heart attack may be passing out. When the reason an older person passed out cannot be pinpointed, an EKG may provide evidence to suggest a heart attack or heart rhythm disturbance. Such persons need to be hospitalized immediately because of the high risk of sudden death.

In other cases, passing out may be the first sign of pneumonia or a serious urinary infection (see Chapter 20). Older persons often do not develop a fever or other common signs of pneumonia, such as a cough, the way younger persons usually do.

Another common cause of passing out is dehydration. Older persons who have not been eating well may become so dehydrated that their blood pressure falls markedly and they pass out. Of course, the question of *why* they stopped eating needs to be addressed. The sudden onset of poor eating is commonly a sign of toxicity from an excess of certain medicines (especially digoxin or Dilantin) or of a developing infection.

In a person who may not have had regular checkups, passing out may be the end result of significant bleeding from the intestines. Often this bleeding occurs very slowly. Under such circumstances it may escape detection until a fall takes place. This fall may be the reason the person was brought to the hospital emergency room. There, a blood count may show anemia (low red blood cell count). Cancer of the right side of the colon is an especially common cause of such anemia. Sometimes such persons have lost as many four or five pints of blood and require a transfusion.

Less Serious Causes of Passing Out

Somewhat—but *only* somewhat—less serious causes of passing out are heart rhythm disturbances and poor circulation to the brain.

Heart Rhythm Disturbances. As the heart gets older, it may develop problems with beating. This can come about as the result of a heart attack—a sudden event—or from clogging of the arteries—a slow and gradual process. When heart rhythm becomes disturbed sufficiently, the heart may begin to beat too slowly, or too quickly; or, it may "skip beats" for several seconds. Whatever the problem, if the heart fails to pump effectively for a long enough period, so little blood gets to the brain that the person passes out. When the rhythm disturbance occurs continuously, the nature of the problem will be apparent by looking at a single EKG tracing. However, when the problem occurs only intermittently, some form of heart monitoring is necessary to detect it. In the more serious cases, the patient is admitted to the hospital, and the heartbeat is monitored on a TV-type screen. In less serious cases, a Holter monitor is hooked up. This is a continuous EKG recording, typically kept for a period of 24 hours. Wires from the machine are attached to the chest over the heart area. The machine is only about the size of a portable cassette recorder. Since it can be strapped on and carried about, patients are often tested while going about their usual business, and do not have to be hospitalized. Unfortunately, not all cases of heart rhythm disturbance are "caught" during the first 24-hour session, so more than one session may be ordered by the doctor—particularly if the person continues to pass out repeatedly for no apparent reason.

Sometimes the heart rhythm problem can be treated with pills. This is often the case when the heart beats very rapidly at times, or skips too many beats in a short interval. In other cases, the heart may suddenly begin beating very slowly—perhaps as slowly as 25 or 30 beats per minute (instead of the usual 60 to 100 per minute). Such cases are often treated by implanting a permanent pacemaker. This machine, slightly smaller than a pack of cigarettes, is surgically placed just beneath the skin—usually near the left shoulder, on the front of the chest. It has wires that are placed so as to travel into a large vein down to the inside of the heart. There, an electrode stimulates the heart to beat at a constant rate—usually 73 beats per minute. The pacemaker is powered by a tiny battery that lasts for years. Recently, it has been suggested that pacemakers are currently being implanted unnecessarily about 20 percent of the time. Although this is a controversial area, it might be wise to consider a second opinion before proceeding when there is any question.

Poor Circulation to the Brain. Poor circulation to the brain often occurs because of clogged arteries in the neck. There are two sets of such arteries: one travels up the back of the neck, the other up the front. The set in the back of the neck are called the vertebral arteries or the vertebral-basilar circulation. These latter arteries are more difficult to treat because they are hard to get at, being surrounded by spinal vertebrae. Often, when no other cause can be found for dizziness or passing out, clogging of the vertebral-basilar circulations, called **vertebral-basilar insufficiency,** is felt to be the cause. The arteries in front of the neck are the two carotid arteries. They are easily photographed with an ultrasound imaging device. This device produces a photograph by bouncing sound waves from the arteries; it requires no injection of dye. When such carotid ultrasound photographs show significant enough narrowing, doctors sometimes operate to remove the obstruction—an operation called **carotid endarterectomy.** However, this is a controversial operation, and doctors often disagree among themselves as to how much obstruction warrants surgery in which patients. As with any operation, it never hurts to get a second opinion when there is any question.

Least Serious Causes of Passing Out

Certain causes of passing out may perhaps be considered "less serious" than those listed above, although they can still cause hip or other fractures and perhaps death from complications. One of the most common is a large drop in blood pressure from standing up too quickly (and not caused by any of the previously mentioned problems, like pneumonia). A major culprit here is the use of certain drugs which affect the heart's ability to pump blood to the brain when changing position. Exhibit 8–1 lists some of the most frequent offenders of this phenomenon, called **postural hypotension.**

The treatment in some cases of postural hypotension may be simply the removal of the offending drug. However, in certain situations this is not possible. Then, other treatments become more important. These include raising the head of the bed 30 degrees and wearing support stockings to prevent too much blood from collecting in the lower legs. Persons with postural hypotension should avoid both standing and sitting for long periods during the day. Mild exercise during the day may help. It is useful for

Exhibit 8–1 Some Drugs That Have the Potential to Cause Postural
           Hypotension

High Blood Pressure Medications:
  nifedipine
  Minipress (prazosin)
  Captopril
  Aldomet
  clonidine
  hydralazine
  reserpine

Sedatives
  chloral hydrate
  barbiturates (Nembutal, Seconal)

Diuretics

Nitroglycerin preparations
  sublingual nitroglycerine
  long-acting skin patches
  longer acting tablets such as Isordil

Antidepressants
  various tricyclic antidepressants such as Elavil, Tofranil, Norpramin, Pamelor

Antipsychotic drugs
  Thorazine
  Mellaril

Anti-Parkinsonian drug
  Sinemet

Drugs for heart rhythm disturbances
  procainamide (including Procan SR)
  disopyramide (Norpace)

---

such persons to keep their legs elevated when sitting down. Use of
a footstool is good, but even better is any method that raises the
legs higher than the level of the heart. Persons with postural
hypotension should avoid very hot baths or showers, as well as
high temperatures, alcohol, and large meals. They should add
extra salt to their food (if this is not forbidden by such conditions
as heart failure or high blood pressure). Coffee after meals may be
helpful in keeping the pressure up at a time when it tends to drop.
In severe cases, certain drugs may be prescribed to make the body
retain fluid, and thereby *increase* the blood pressure. Persons with
postural hypotension should be careful when arising—especially
after lying down for a long time. They should always sit up for
several minutes before standing up.

A harmless cause of passing out—provided no injury occurs—is a fall in blood pressure caused by exaggerated natural reflexes. In some persons this happens after urinating (especially in men with prostate problems), defecating, or during an episode of coughing. Treatment in such cases may be for such men to sit down when urinating, use stool softeners to avoid straining at stool, and use cough-suppressing syrups to prevent prolonged bouts of coughing.

Falls Without Loss of Consciousness

Falls *without* passing out can arise from the same conditions which cause the person to *both* pass out *and* fall down. For example, heart rhythm disturbances that are not serious enough to cause passing out may still cause temporary wooziness and loss of balance. The same is true of pneumonia or a drop in standing blood pressure from drugs. In addition, other problems can cause loss of balance but do not cause loss of consciousness.

Eye Problems. Many normal changes in vision make it more likely that an older person will fall. Adjusting to a darkened room takes older persons longer. Depth perception is less accurate. Color discrimination declines. In addition, vision may be reduced. Other causes of reduced vision include cataracts, glaucoma, and macular degeneration (see Chapter 13). Many people do not realize that some strokes cause blindness in certain directions, such as to the right or to the left in each eye. Thus, persons who have had strokes may be unable to see objects in their paths, putting them at high risk for tripping and falling down.

Hearing Problems. The gradual decline in hearing that comes with age may increase the likelihood of accidents because of failure to detect warning noises. Combined with poor vision, such older persons are at much higher risk for falling when out in public.

Dizziness. Dizziness may have a large variety of causes. High blood pressure is actually an infrequent one, although many people who become dizzy fear that it is caused by their blood pressure getting too high. Persons who have been alcoholics for many years and persons with vitamin B-12 deficiency may lose their ability to place their feet properly when walking; and this may cause a feeling similar to dizziness. Vitamin B-12 deficiency becomes more common in later years. It is especially common in persons who have had part of their stomachs removed. It can cause the red blood cells to become larger—something detectable by the doctor when a complete blood count is done. Since vitamin B-12 deficiency commonly occurs in persons whose stomach has lost the ability to absorb it, it can only be properly given to such persons in injection form, in order to bypass the stomach. (Vitamin B-12 is sold over the counter in oral form, but it cannot provide much benefit to such persons.)

Vertigo. Vertigo differs from dizziness in that persons who experience vertigo feel a sense of *motion*, such as the room spinning around or themselves spinning. Sometimes the cause may be a virus that attacks the balance center, located in the inner ear. The sensation of vertigo usually begins suddenly and typically lasts for only a day or two, although it may persist for a few weeks or longer. Sudden changes of position, such as lying down quickly, sitting up quickly, or turning the head quickly, can worsen the sensation when the attack is full blown. The virus may follow a head cold or flu or pneumonia. Various drugs, such as motion sickness and antinausea pills, are used to treat the condition. Poor circulation to the brain from the vertebral-basilar circulation at the back of the neck (mentioned earlier in this chapter) can produce vertigo in older persons. Vertigo from this cause is usually of brief duration; but it can recur frequently.

Hypothermia. An important cause of falls in olders persons is hypothermia, or low body temperature, perhaps from inadequate heating. Older persons tend not to tolerate cold temperatures as well as younger persons. An ideal gift for an older person is a blanket or a sweater.

Balance Problems. With advancing age, many normal reflexes slow, and the ability to keep one's balance is reduced. This can lead to falls. However, with certain conditions, balance difficulties become greatly increased. One of the more common is Parkinson's disease, which ultimately affects one person in 50 (see Chapter 16).

Mobility Problems

Although the previous problems can cause dramatic and sudden inability to keep one's balance, falls by older people may also be the result of gradual deterioration of the muscles and bones.

Various kinds of arthritis can make movement so painful that the person tends to become inactive. The inactivity, in turn, causes the muscles to shrink with lack of use. The aphorism "use it or lose it" summarizes the basic principle here. It is important for older persons to keep active in order to preserve their ability to get about. In severe cases, the help of a physical therapist or a family member may be needed to keep some persons mobile, so that they can continue to perform the usual activities of daily living. Exercise programs may concentrate on various areas, according to the needs of the individual. Certain muscles—particularly those thigh muscles which straighten the leg—may need to be strengthened. Endurance may be another goal. Coordination and balance may be problem areas, especially in getting out of bed, standing up from a chair, and turning around. If there are stairs in the home, it may be important for the aide or therapist to emphasize special exercises for stair climbing. Stretching and range-of-motion exercises may be needed. Active range of motion (the patient moving the arm or leg voluntarily) is used when possible. Extremely weakened persons may be capable of only passive range of motion, in which another person provides all the energy to move the arm or leg. In such weakened persons, range of motion exercises are important to prevent the development of **contractures,** in which arms or legs that are no longer used become "folded up" and stiff, until they can no longer be straightened out.

Safety Measures in the Home

In order to reduce the chances of a fall, certain safety measures can be addressed in the home. Lack of proper eyeglasses is an important start. Proper shoes (no high heels) and clothing (pantlegs should not drag on the ground) are also important. Because of reduced vision, adequate lighting is important, especially on stairways. Both sides of the stairway should have handrails that are long enough to allow the person to get completely to the bottom while still holding on. Light switches should be at both the top and bottom of stairs. The top and bottom steps—particularly the bottom step, where most falls in the home take place—should be painted in bright, contrasting colors, or lined with bright tape.

In bedrooms, light switches should be reachable from the doorway. Nightlights should be provided to completely illuminate the path between the bathroom and the bedroom. Slippery surfaces are dangerous. They can have various causes. Polished wax floors are a known hazard; nonslipping wax can be used instead. Carpets and throw rugs should have all edges taped to the floor or tacked down. Kitchen mats should be nonskid. Kitchen cabinets should be within easy reach. If not, proper stepladders should be available, so the person does not have to stand on a chair. Reaching tongs may be needed. In the kitchen, all pilot lights on a gas stove should be working properly. In the bathroom (especially in the tub or shower) and on stairs, there should be skid-proof strips.

Clutter should be avoided—especially on stairs. Loose electrical cords on the floor are a common hazard. They should be tightly secured against the wall. Low chairs should be removed, or firm pillows placed to effectively raise their height. All chairs should have sufficiently long armrests that they can be used for support when standing up. A raised toilet seat may be needed in the bathroom. Outside the home, all steps should be well repaired, handrails secure, and sidewalks even and in good repair. There should be adequate lighting here, as well.

Management of Mobility Problems

Mobility in the elderly varies along a continuum. At one extreme are those who are independently ambulatory without having to use any assistive devices. At the other extreme are those who are completely bedbound. Near the active end of this spectrum are those who can get about on their own, but suffer from joint pains and stiffness, particularly in the mornings and especially during cold weather. These joint problems are more troublesome when they occur in the weight-bearing joints (the hips, knees, and ankles), and the lower back. (Treatment of joint pains and stiffness is discussed in Chapter 10.)

Persons with more serious mobility problems may need devices to assist them. Such devices vary from the simple cane to the quad-cane (a cane that branches out at the bottom to four "feet"), to walkers of varying types (some have wheels; others are the stationary, "pick-up" type). Patients no longer able to walk should be kept in a sitting position as much as possible each day to prevent pneumonia. Patients who are too heavy for a single caregiver to lift out of bed require a Hoyer lift to accomplish the transfer. Although used in hospitals and nursing homes, it can also be brought into the home. It is a kind of miniature crane that works on the same principle as a tire jack. A canvas is placed under the patient, and the ends attached to the "jaws" of the lift, which is cranked to move the patient out of bed and into a wheelchair. Although not particularly complex, learning to use it can nevertheless prove to be a more ambitious undertaking than many families bargain for when they envision home care.

Other important maneuvers for the debilitated, home-bound patient are:

- transferring to the sitting-up position in bed from the lying position;
- transferring to the standing position from the sitting position;
- walking varying distances on a level surface, with or without a device; and
- climbing stairs inside the home.

Physical therapists can come into the home to assist the caregiver in techniques for accomplishing the above transfers. They also can train the patient with exercises to increase strength and endurance for transfers, walking, and stair-climbing. As debilitated patients approach the status of being bedbound, the potential for bedsores looms dramatically (see Chapter 21).

A variety of devices can do much to "make life easier"—and safer—for those intent on staying in the home in spite of mobility limitations:

- bedside commode
- hospital bed (mechanical or electric)
- wheelchair
- tub or shower chair
- handrails in the hallways and the bathroom—especially by the toilet and inside the tub and shower areas.

Medicare will pay for many of these devices with a prescription from the doctor, as long as the prescription lists the appropriate diagnosis.

Chapter 9

OSTEOPOROSIS

Osteoporosis is a condition of generalized bone loss throughout the body. Although the bones may shrink in size, of far more importance is the fact that they become less dense and therefore more brittle. Osteoporosis has been called a "silent" disease because it develops slowly and insidiously, giving no symptoms until far advanced. Often, by the time it is diagnosed, much damage has been done and the person is at high risk for breaking bones. The bones most subject to fracture from osteoporosis are in the wrists, hips, and spine. Primarily through complications from broken hips, osteoporosis has been pegged as the 12th leading cause of death in the United States.

The Significance of Bone Loss

The strength of bone is proportional to the square of its density. Thus, bone which is twice as dense is four times as strong. Conversely, bone which has lost half its mass is only one-fourth as strong. This is why women who suffer from severe osteoporosis have been known to break backbones through the mere act of sneezing or coughing, and to suffer broken hips with only minor stresses, such as stepping down from a curb.

The main ingredient of bone is calcium. We are taught that we need calcium the most during the early years of our life, when we are growing up and getting taller. While it is true that young people do need calcium for growing bones, many people fail to realize that our need for calcium does not stop once our bones have reached their full length. Many older women especially don't get enough calcium to prevent osteoporosis.

The loss of bone begins around age 40. Bone loss occurs both on the outer surface and deep inside the supporting structures of the bone. While both parts of the bone are important, the supporting structures are relatively more important. Women lose up to about 60 percent of these supporting structures; men, up to about 40 percent. After some 30 years of this process, women may have only half as much bone in their body as during their peak years.

Immediately after menopause, women suddenly begin to lose bone quite rapidly. During the first five to ten years—and especially during the first five years—women lose bone about five times faster than they do later on. However, even in later years, women still lose about 1 to 2 percent of their bone mass each year.

Who Is Likely to Develop Osteoporosis?

Having the condition of osteoporosis is usually defined by having broken a bone without the kind of injury that normally would cause such a break. By this definition, about one in every four women develops osteoporosis. Another definition of osteoporosis is based on bone density. Below a certain density level, 90 percent of crushed backbones have been found to take place without any obvious injury. By this definition, half of all women over 65 and all women over 85 have osteoporosis of the spine.

Women are about eight times more likely than men to develop osteoporosis. Part of the reason is that men exercise more, start off with greater bone and muscle mass, and consume more foods that are high in calcium. Certain other factors increase the chances that one will get osteoporosis, among them the following:

- Caucasian or Oriental race, and especially northern European ancestry
- family history of relatives with osteoporosis
- height less than 5-½ feet
- thin frame
- low body weight
- light-colored hair
- freckles
- not having borne any children (if female)

- not having breast-fed (if female)
- advanced age: after menopause in females; after 65 in males; and increasing with age
- early menopause, or hysterectomy before menopause
- low-calcium diet
- diet high in protein or coffee (three or more cups per day)
- cigarette smoking
- alcoholism
- inactivity

Obese people are less likely to develop osteoporosis, probably because fatty tissues convert certain hormones produced by the adrenal glands and by the ovaries into estrogen, and estrogen tends to prevent osteoporosis.

Evaluating Suspected Osteoporosis

There are no early physical signs that osteoporosis has begun. By the time one is able to notice the physical changes osteoporosis brings, it will already have reached a relatively advanced stage. The signs of advanced osteoporosis are a loss of height and curvature of the upper back. Loss of height can be gauged by measuring one's arm span (the distance from the tips of the fingers of one hand to the tips of the fingers of the other, with the hands held outstretched), as well as height. Except in black persons, the arm span equals one's height after growth has peaked. If your arm span is now more than your height, you may have begun to lose bone in your spine from osteoporosis.

In evaluating a person with suspected osteoporosis, the doctor takes a complete history, performs a physical examination, and may order a battery of blood and urine tests. (If the tests are normal, that does not mean the person cannot have osteoporosis; the tests are done primarily to look for unusual causes of osteoporosis.)

Regular x-rays cannot detect bone loss until it has become relatively advanced. To more fully evaluate osteoporosis, or its response to treatment, doctors measure bone density. This is done with special machines that pass gamma rays through the wrists, spine, or hips. Patients concerned about radiation will be reassured to know that the exposure of this test is only one-tenth as much as with a standard chest x-ray. Doctors who evaluate their patients with bone density measurements sometimes begin with a "baseline" measurement of women at age 45, and repeat the measurement within two years after their periods have stopped. Such measurements may be especially helpful to women who are undecided about whether to begin estrogen treatment to prevent osteoporosis. A potential disadvantage is that valuable time is lost (in the case of women with osteoporosis) if one does not begin estrogen therapy immediately after periods stop, since that is when bone loss is heaviest. Unfortunately, we do not yet have a good way to know in advance who will develop osteoporosis. The best doctors can now do is guess which persons are *most likely* to get osteoporosis—based on the risk factors mentioned earlier—and urge them to take preventive measures.

The Effects of Osteoporosis

The ultimate effects of osteoporosis are manifested by fractures and by bone loss in certain areas, such as the mouth and the spine. Just where and how often fractures occur was discussed in Chapter 8.

Bone loss from osteoporosis occurs in the bones that normally support teeth (the aveolar ridges). Too much bone loss here makes it impossible for dentures to be worn properly. This in turn, leads to chewing problems, poor nutrition, and a change in appearance (see Chapter 15).

The gradual effects of osteoporosis over a period of decades results in shortening and curvature of the upper spine into what has come to be known as **dowager's hump.** In severe cases, the distortion can be so severe as to interfere with breathing. In such cases, the compressed lung is pushed downward, making the abdomen protrude. Persons with dowager's hump often suffer from back pains as the backbones progressively collapse.

The Importance of Prevention

Knowing how to prevent osteoporosis requires a basic understanding of the content of bone. Bone consists primarily of calcium and phosphate compounds. It is virtually impossible not to get enough phosphate in the diet. However, insufficient calcium intake commonly begins after age 14 in females and becomes slightly worse year after year until menopause. At menopause, insufficient calcium intake in women suddenly becomes more marked, on the average. Certain medications can affect dietary calcium. Antacids which contain aluminum (almost all of them) interfere with absorption of calcium. In addition, most antacids, as well as milk of magnesia, contain compounds that tend to deplete phosphates from the body. They therefore have the potential to cause bone loss if used excessively.

Prevention is by far preferable to waiting until osteoporosis has manifested itself. Then, it is often too late to do much. Prevention of osteoporosis is accomplished by attention to diet, exercise, and good posture, and frequently by the use of calcium supplements, vitamin D, and estrogen replacement therapy (for women). Although smoking and excessive drinking have been associated with osteoporosis, we do not know precisely how much these habits relate to this condition. No studies of osteoporosis have yet been done of smokers or alcoholics who gave up their habits.

Diet, Exercise, and Good Posture

Diet. The subject of diet in the prevention of osteoporosis is discussed in Chapter 22, which emphasizes the importance of adequate calcium intake. A list of calcium-rich foods is provided in Appendix C.

Exercise. Prolonged bed rest causes rapid bone loss. A similar phenomenon has been observed in astronauts floating weightlessly in space. Conversely, daily exercise, especially of the weight-bearing sort, tends to preserve bone. A half-hour walk every day is also recommended. Swimming is less beneficial for bone stimulation, since it does not involve weight bearing. Sports that are ideal for stimulating bone growth are running, bicycle riding, and tennis. The minimum amount of exercise should be 30 minutes three times a week (see Chapter 25 for further information).

Good Posture. Good posture is important in preventing curvature of the spine from osteoporosis. When sitting, it is best to use a straight chair with a high back. And, the lower back can be supported by a pillow. Avoid craning the neck forward when in the sitting position. When standing, keep the back straight, the head held high, shoulders back, and chin in. The feet should be kept pointed straight ahead. When lifting heavy objects, it is important to keep the back as vertical as possible, rather than bending over. Lifting should be done primarily with the leg muscles, and not with the back. When lying down, a way of keeping the spine straight is to have one pillow under the head and one or two pillows resting behind the knees.

Calcium Supplements

Older women need at least 1,200 to 1,500 mg of calcium per day. Since it is hard to get this much calcium in one's diet, it is often necessary to take calcium tablets. Diets high in calcium also tend to raise cholesterol, because most high-calcium foods, such as dairy products, also happen to be high in saturated fats. Therefore, persons who try to reduce cholesterol usually end up reducing their calcium intake. One way around this dilemma is to take calcium supplements.

The use of calcium supplements has been found to reduce fractures of the spine by one-half. Although doctors can tell in retrospect whether an older woman likely did not get enough calcium in earlier years, there is not yet any test which can reassure an older woman taking calcium supplements that she is taking enough.

Caution About Calcium Supplements. Although calcium supplements are available without a prescription, taking too much calcium may be harmful, especially if you take in more than twice as much as you need. One risk of excess calcium intake is the milk-alkali syndrome (discussed in Chapter 17). Persons who have had kidney or urinary tract stones may need special urine tests before calcium tablets are considered.

How to Take Calcium Supplements. Half of the daily dose should be taken at bedtime, since it is believed that calcium is absorbed better overnight. The rest should be taken before meals. Most calcium tablets contain from 250 to 500 mg of elemental calcium. It is important to remember that calcium requirements mentioned are elemental calcium, not the total amount of compound. There are a number of forms of calcium on the market. The most common are calcium carbonate, calcium phosphate, calcium lactate, and calcium gluconate. These contain various percentages of *elemental* calcium. Respectively, their percentages are 40, 31, 13, and 9 percent. This means that one can take in a higher amount of elemental calcium with fewer pills by choosing a calcium carbonate compound (such as Os-Cal). However, calcium carbonate tends to cause intestinal problems such as "gas" in some persons. Calcium gluconate and calcium lactate are easier to digest. Calcium citrate is of value for persons who have had part of their stomachs removed surgically and therefore do not absorb calcium as well due to having less stomach acid. It is also better for persons who tend to form kidney stones. Certain calcium preparations, such as dolomite and bone meal, are not recommended because they may be contaminated with lead or other toxic metals.

It is important to drink plenty of liquids if you are taking calcium tablets, to minimize your chances of getting kidney stones. (However, kidney stones only rarely develop in persons who have never had them before.)

Certain types of diuretics ("water pills"), such as Lasix, tend to increase the calcium level in the urine, and therefore increase the risk of kidney stones in persons taking calcium tablets. Other types of water pills (such as hydrochlorthiazide) that are commonly used to treat high blood pressure tend to *prevent* loss of calcium through the kidneys.

Vitamin D Supplements

Vitamin D is important in the absorption of calcium. Most multi-vitamin tablets contain 400 international units (IU), which is a sufficient daily amount. In the United States, most milk has 400 IU of vitamin D added to each quart. Foods high in vitamin D are liver and egg yolks. However, these foods are extremely high in cholesterol as well. Persons who get a lot of sunlight every day may not need to take vitamin D supplements, since the effect of sunlight on the skin produces vitamin D naturally in the body.

Vitamin D can be toxic when taken in relatively large doses. Although doctors do commonly prescribe doses of 50 to 100 thousand units for patients with certain hormone disorders, this can lead to toxicity in some cases. To be on the safe side, no more than 1,000 units daily should be taken without being under a doctor's supervision.

Estrogen

For women who have reached the menopause, or who have had their menopause early because of a hysterectomy, the most effective measure for preventing osteoporosis is to use estrogen replacement therapy (available only with a doctor's prescription) until at least age 70. After age 70, the use of estrogens is more controversial, because of the side effect of an increased risk of blood clots in the very old. We do not understand exactly how and why estrogen helps prevent osteoporosis, but we do know that it does help—in fact, even more than increased calcium intake. Estrogen also improves the cholesterol profile, even though it slightly elevates the amount of fat in the blood. The net effect is believed to be a slight beneficial effect on heart disease.

Cautions About the Use of Estrogen. Estrogen should not be taken by women who have had breast cancer. Nor should it be taken by women with fibrocystic breasts because they have a greater risk of breast cancer if they take estrogen. Estrogen, given alone, increases the risk of cancer of the lining of the uterus (endometrium). Women who have had a hysterectomy do not have to worry about this, since they no longer have a uterus. Some sources say that women who take estrogen have a five to ten times higher risk of developing endometrial cancer. However, this risk can be avoided if another female hormone, progesterone, is also given during part of the monthly cycle. The use of both estrogen and progesterone each month in a cyclic fashion may actually reduce the risk of breast cancer, as well as cancer of the lining of the uterus, according to some recent studies.

Other women who are advised *not* to take estrogen hormones are those who have had problems with blood clots in their veins, migraine headaches, a history of liver disease, or diabetes. Women who have benign fibroid tumors of the uterus should also avoid estrogen because estrogen may make these tumors grow larger. Estrogen use can also lead to increased blood pressure and gallstones. A history of any abnormal bleeding, varicose veins, or high blood pressure may be reason not to take estrogen.

Occasionally, estrogen has also been known to produce large vascular tumors in the liver. Though rather rare, these tumors are dangerous in that they can rupture spontaneously or with minor injury and cause severe internal bleeding.

Less serious consequences of estrogen use are breast tenderness and fluid retention. The most common side effect of estrogen is nausea. All women who are taking estrogen, or any female hormones, after the menopause should have thorough, periodic gynecological examinations.

How Estrogen Is Given.   When female hormones are given to women who still have their uterus, a typical—but not the only— regimen is for estrogen (such as Premarin 0.625 mg) to be taken the first 25 days of the month, and for medroxyprogesterone (such as Provera 10 mg) to be taken from days 16 through 25 each month. During the remaining days of the month neither drug is taken. This therapy generally continues for a least 10 years. Some doctors believe that virtually all the benefits of estrogen therapy are quickly lost soon after the woman stops taking it, and are adamantly opposed to such a "short" course. Such doctors believe that estrogen therapy should continue for life, despite the view of others (mentioned earlier in this chapter) that there is a greater likelihood of side effects in the very old. Most women who are placed on cyclic estrogen and progesterone each month will begin having periods again. This does not indicate a return of fertility, and is of no consequence.

Treatment of Osteoporosis

Once osteoporosis has developed, it is difficult to reverse the bone loss that has already occurred. Aside from treatment of specific fractures, little can be done to strengthen existing bones. To date, no effective treatment to reverse osteoporosis has yet been approved by the Food and Drug Administration.

Women with osteoporosis are advised to wear low-heeled shoes with soft soles and foam or other cushion inserts.

Chapter 10

ARTHRITIS

Arthritis afflicts more senior citizens than any other chronic condition: 57 percent of women and 36 percent of men. The first thing many people think of when arthritis is mentioned is the gnarled hands of people with advanced **rheumatoid arthritis**—the crippling kind. Relatively few senior citizens are afflicted with rheumatoid arthritis—somewhere from 7.5 to 25 percent. Although there are about 100 different kinds of arthritis, the vast majority of people over 65 who have arthritis suffer from the ordinary type, called **osteoarthritis.** Also called "degenerative joint disease," it comes just from getting old, although injuries and overuse of joints accelerate its progress. Another important type of arthritis, which increasingly strikes with advancing age, is **gout.**

Rheumatoid Arthritis: The Crippling Kind of Arthritis

An "Inflammation" of the Joints

Although the word arthritis literally means, "inflammation of the joint," the ordinary type of arthritis—osteoarthritis—would more accurately be characterized as a "wearing out" of the joint. In contrast, rheumatoid arthritis is truly more of an "inflammation" of the joint. It damages the joint lining and cartilage and also causes inflammation in tendons, ligaments, and even bone. Although rheumatoid arthritis most typically affects the joints, it is a disease of the entire body; it can cause weakness, poor appetite, and

89

occasionally even fever and night sweats. Although it has sometimes been difficult for doctors to decide just when a person could
be said to have actual "rheumatoid arthritis," the American Rheu-
matism Association recently made the diagnosis easier by revising
its criteria for the first time since 1958. Now, instead of a person
being able to be classified as having "probable" rheumatoid arthritis, persons with joint disease are deemed either to have rheumatoid arthritis or not. To have rheumatoid arthritis, a person must
have at least four of the following:

- morning stiffness lasting at least an hour
- swelling in at least three joints
- swelling of the hands
- symmetrical swelling
- abnormal x-rays of the hands typical of rheumatoid arthritis
- typical rheumatoid nodules, which come just below the surface
  of the skin
- a positive blood test for the "rheumatoid factor" (present in 95
  percent of cases)

After age 60 rheumatoid arthritis afflicts women more than men
in a ratio of 4 to 1. It should be emphasized that rheumatoid
arthritis tends to be a much more serious disease than the ordinary
type of arthritis. Estimates are that 20 percent of people with
rheumatoid arthritis die from it, and another 20 percent die from
the complications of being treated for it. Persons with diagnosed
rheumatoid arthritis must undergo treatment for the disease as
soon as it is discovered; otherwise the inflammation to the joints is
more damaging.

Treatment of Rheumatoid Arthritis

The usual treatment of rheumatoid arthritis is no different from
the treatment of most other types of arthritis (joint inflammation),
and consists of either aspirin or the so-called "nonsteroidal anti-
inflammatory agents" (NSAIs). Other means of treatment include
salves, cortisone, weight loss, and physical therapy.

Aspirin.   For those who can tolerate it, aspirin is the cheapest
and often the most effective treatment. Up to three of the standard
size (325 mg) aspirin taken four times a day commonly may be
needed and is not excessive in most cases. However, one should

gradually work up to this many pills and use only as many as necessary. Some arthritis patients need more aspirin, but higher doses are accompanied by a greater risk of side effects. A classical symptom of aspirin toxicity is ringing in the ears. Some people suffer bleeding tendencies (such as bleeding gums) at much lower doses—two or even one aspirin a day. So-called "arthritis-strength" formulas of aspirin merely have a larger dose of aspirin and offer no advantage over taking a larger quantity of regular-strength aspirin. Regular-strength aspirin is 325 mg.

NSAIs. For those not able to tolerate aspirin, one of the NSAIs (nonsteroidal anti-inflammatory agents) is often prescribed. The best-known drug in this category is ibuprofen. It became available over the counter not long ago in the 200 mg size. Some of the better-known over-the-counter brands are Advil, Medipren, and Nuprin.

Like aspirin, NSAIs also can cause upset stomach in some people. But they are much *less* irritating to the stomach, in general, than aspirin. A side effect not present in aspirin is a minor degree of fluid retention, but this is rarely much of a problem. In prescription strength, the best-known brand of ibuprofen is Motrin. It is currently available in sizes which range from 300 to 800 mg. The maximum dose generally prescribed is about 800 mg three times a day.

Trying to review the individual NSAIs is like trying to review the movies. It is hard to know which will please which people. I confess to favoring Motrin, Naprosyn, and Feldene. Feldene is one of the most expensive per tablet, but only needs to be taken once a day.

Salves. Various salves for arthritis exert their action through skin irritants, which increase blood flow to the skin for brief periods of time. This produces redness and warmth to the skin, but has minimal, if any, effect on underlying joints. Such products are absorbed through the skin and may produce side effects if overused.

Cortisone. If aspirin and NSAIs fail, sometimes cortisone is injected into a joint, a treatment that may give relief for several weeks or months. Occasionally, cortisone is given by mouth for a few weeks; the side effects of cortisone begin to mount if given for much longer, and in such cases its use is generally considered "a last resort."

Besides cortisone, numerous other drug treatments for rheumatoid arthritis are popular, including the injection of gold salts into the joint; but detailing these is beyond the scope of this book. However, general measures that are useful for any type of chronic arthritis are weight loss (in overweight persons) and physical therapy.

Losing Weight. In the case of weight-bearing joints (hips, knees, and ankles, especially), it is most important for obese persons to lose weight. Many orthopedic surgeons are reluctant to perform hip or knee surgery for arthritic conditions until obese patients have first brought their weight under control.

Physical Therapy. It is very important, especially in severe cases, to perform daily exercises for flexibility and strengthening in the affected joints. Alternating periods of rest with periods of exercise is important. One should be careful not to exercise affected joints too much. Various types of heat treatment (such as hot packs and immersion into warm wax) are often helpful. In other cases, cold packs are helpful. Some persons benefit from alternating heat and cold treatments.

Osteoarthritis: The Common Kind of Arthritis

A "Wearing Out" of the Joints

Osteoarthritis, the ordinary type of arthritis, does not usually cause as much inflammation of the joints as does rheumatoid arthritis. It afflicts almost everybody to some degree in later life and becomes more common with increasing age. Almost 90 percent of people suffer from it to some degree after age 60. In most cases it is a mild disease, but sometimes it can be disabling. The cause is not known; nor is there a cure or any known way to stop the progress of the disease. It is characterized mainly by pain and stiffness in various joints—some tend to be affected more than others. In the hands, osteoarthritis tends to affect the joints at the *ends* of the fingers, whereas rheumatoid arthritis tends to affect the finger joints that are closer to the wrists. The joint stiffness is typically brief—a half hour or less, in contrast to rheumatoid arthritis. Stiffness tends to occur after rest. Pain is not much of a problem until the disease is advanced. Osteoarthritis commonly affects the neck, the lower back, the hips, and the knees. Often x-rays are used to determine the degree of joint damage.

Treatment of Osteoarthritis

The treatment of osteoarthritis is the same as the treatment of rheumatoid arthritis with respect to the use of aspirin, NSAIs, salves, weight loss, and physical therapy. Cortisone tablets and cortisone joint injections are also used in the case of severe inflammation, though this is less common because osteoarthritis tends to cause less severe inflammation than the rheumatoid type of arthritis. Nevertheless, severe joint damage does occasionally occur in patients with osteoarthritis. When all else fails, surgery is often helpful here. In the early stages of osteoarthritis, surgeons sometimes clear out debris and smooth joint surfaces, a procedure known as **debridement**. When joint surfaces are misaligned (usually in the knee joint), the joint surfaces may be cut to bring them into better alignment, a procedure known as **osteotomy. Fusion** may be performed on joints to relieve pain or provide support—a procedure most often done in the cervical or lumbar spine. **Total joint replacement** may be performed on very badly damaged hip or knee joints. Such total joint replacement, in general, is more successful in the case of hips than with knees.

Gout: Another Kind of Arthritis

The "Disease of Kings"

Gout has been called "the disease of kings" because in centuries past only kings could afford the kinds of rich foods—steaks, shellfish, alcohol, and rich desserts—that are linked to gout. Foods high in compounds called *purines* are broken down by the body into uric acid. It is the crystallization of uric acid into one or more joints which causes this very painful inflammatory disease. Although fairly uncommon, especially in young people, gout tends to occur more frequently with advancing age. The reason is that older persons often begin to suffer some degree of decline in kidney function, and this results in less clearing out of uric acid from the bloodstream. When a high uric acid level results in crystallization into a joint, about half the time that joint is the big toe. Gout typically comes on rapidly, within a period of a few hours, and the pain is so excruciating that it is typical for even the touch of a bedsheet to be intolerable. In addition to the marked tenderness, there is heat, swelling, and redness of the affected joint. Occasionally, several joints can be affected at once.

Gout goes away by itself within a few days to a few weeks, even if untreated. However, the symptoms are so severe that medical treatment is usually sought. Although most gout is due to the combination of heredity, old age, and following the wrong diet (one high in purines), certain "water pills" (the thiazide diuretics, such as hydrochlorthiazide) tend to raise the uric acid level and can sometimes bring on an attack.

The average age when gout first strikes is 52, and 95 percent of cases happen to men. However, because it is often difficult to prove that a person has gout (the current definition requires finding uric acid crystals in joint fluid), it has been suspected that a large number of older women suffer from it. At least, it has been found that they respond to treatment for certain attacks of arthritis as if they had gout. More research needs to be done in this area.

Treatment of Gout

When medical treatment for gout is sought because of severe pain from inflammation caused by excessive levels of uric acid in the blood and consequent crystallization of uric acid in one or more joints, the drug colchicine can often bring relief in a few hours. In its "full course," it is given as often as every hour up to about 6 tablets per day or 10 tablets per week. Colchicine, however, can produce toxic effects—nausea, vomiting, diarrhea, and stomach cramps—and there is no way to know when a toxic level has been reached until the symptoms begin. For this reason, the full course of colchicine is seldom given to older persons; and many doctors avoid using colchicine at all in this age group, choosing instead to treat gout attacks with one of the NSAIs. The powerful NSAI Indocin (a brand of indomethacin) is commonly used for this purpose. However, Indocin is harsher on the stomach than most other NSAIs, and (like other NSAIs, but more so) has been known occasionally to cause sudden decline in kidney function—a dangerous condition that usually reverses itself once the drug is stopped. When Indocin or other drugs that may upset the stomach must be given, this side effect can often be anticipated and prevented by first giving drugs that can calm the stomach (for details, see Chapter 17).

A person who has suffered an attack of gout should avoid foods that are high in purines (see Appendix F). People who get recurrent gout attacks are often placed on long-term daily therapy with colchicine, allopurinol or Benemid, or a combination of colchicine and Benemid known as Colbenemid. Benemid, however, can *bring on* an attack of gout if begun at too high a dose, or too soon after an attack.

Sexuality and Arthritis

Many older persons with advanced arthritis, especially rheumatoid arthritis, abandon pursuance of an active sex life. However, the judicious use of some of the above treatments, taking a warm bath, and adjustments in body positions and timing of sexual activity, such as resting beforehand and avoiding the early morning hours when joint stiffness is especially bad, can enable most arthritics to continue to enjoy a normal and satisfying sex life.

Chapter 11

DIABETES

The term **diabetes** generally refers to diabetes *mellitus*, a serious disease which affects many Americans, young and old alike.* Also called **sugar diabetes**, it is a disorder in which the body does not properly handle dextro-glucose (later referred to as D-glucose), a common sugar. All cells require glucose, and without it they will not function. Brain cells particularly sustain rapid and sometimes permanent damage when deprived of glucose for very long.

Glucose is carried to the various cells of the body through the bloodstream. It enters with the aid of a hormone called insulin, which is secreted by the pancreas. When the pancreas does not produce enough insulin or the insulin for various reasons cannot be used properly, glucose builds up in the bloodstream and eventually spills into the urine. It is when the blood levels of glucose rise to dangerously high levels that the three classic symptoms of diabetes occur: **excessive thirst and drinking, excessive urination (not just frequent urination but frequent urination of large quantities), and excessive hunger,† with overeating.**

Diabetes can be controlled. When there is insufficient insulin, some diabetics require periodic (usually once a day) injections of synthetic insulin or insulin that has been extracted from animals. These people are said to be **insulin-dependent**. When the disease is milder, it can often be treated by dietary changes or by pills that stimulate the pancreas to produce more insulin. Generally, diabe-

---

*Technically speaking, there is another, rare, type of diabetes—diabetes *insipidus*—which is also characterized by excessive urination, but without sugar in the urine, and without excessive sugar in the blood. It is a disorder of the pituitary, a gland at the base of skull.
†A late sign, seen only in advanced diabetes which is not controlled.

tes that begins after age 40 is of this type and is often referred to as **adult onset diabetes**. Most children, and many adults under age 40 who become diabetic, are insulin-dependent. And even though the majority of adults over age 40 do not require insulin, some do, and others will eventually need insulin in their later years.

Heredity plays a small role in diabetes, being dwarfed by the factor of obesity in adult onset diabetes. Even when both parents are diabetic, only about 3 to 12 percent of children become diabetic.

Diabetes occurs in 17 percent of persons aged 60 to 74. Another 10 percent have "impaired glucose tolerance," meaning they "fail" a glucose tolerance test (discussed below), but have no signs or symptoms of diabetes. Some of them may eventually develop diabetes.

Untreated diabetics often suffer from weakness and fatigue. There may be fungal rashes in the skin folds of obese persons and vaginal yeast infections (in women). Some diabetics suffer from generalized itching, especially at night. Bruises and cuts tend to heal slowly. Less often, there may be blurred vision, dizziness, headaches, dry skin, and occasionally vomiting and abdominal cramps.

Complications of Diabetes

After 20 or more years of being diabetic, many persons are faced with a host of complications which mainly result from accelerated hardening of the arteries or damage to various nerves. Damage to the back of the eyes (the retinas) tends to come relatively early, with about 50 percent of diabetics being afflicted to a mild or moderate degree after 20 years. However, modern advances in laser surgery have done much to reduce the threat of blindness in diabetics who suffer from eye problems. Reduced vision to the point of blindness reaches its peak after 30 years. Significant degrees of kidney failure begin to affect about 40 percent of diabetics after 30 years. Clogging of the arteries to the feet and legs affects only 20 percent during the first 35 years, but rises dramatically to plague almost 60 percent after 40 years. A late complication of diabetes is disease of the nerves to the feet, causing loss of sensation. Coupled with clogging of the arteries in the legs, this can lead to a variety of foot problems, which are discussed later in the chapter.

Some Long-Term Problems of Diabetics

In addition to the complications just discussed, diabetics can have a host of other problems in the long term, including the following.

Dental Problems. Diabetics are especially susceptible to periodontal disease. Therefore, it is particularly important for them to practice good dental hygiene.

Heart Problems. Diabetics have an increased risk of heart attacks and angina. The nerves which control the heart rate are affected, so that diabetics typically have a faster resting pulse of 90 to 100. Nerves which control the blood pressure cause some diabetics to suffer a large drop in pressure when they first stand up.

Blindness. Eyesight damage is worse than in most other eye diseases because it tends to come on suddenly and leave the person with less vision than is the case with other eye diseases. Although blindness affects only a small percentage of diabetics, many suffer reading difficulty because of swelling in the macular area.

Eye Muscle Paralysis. Diabetes can cause drooping of one of the upper eyelids. It can also typically cause one eye to turn inward and upward. This results in double vision, but almost always lasts less than two months.

Facial Muscle Paralysis. Sometimes there is a temporary paralysis of the muscles on one side of the face. However, there is usually complete recovery.

The Digestive System. There may be slow or unpredictable digestion of food. In the small bowel, nerve damage can cause watery diarrhea which comes mostly at night and which is sometimes associated with fecal incontinence.

Muscle Weakness. Muscle weakness may strike the lower legs especially, followed by the hands. Diabetics may lose the ability to separate their toes. This and other weaknesses typically lead to claw or hammertoe development. In the hands, the grip becomes weak.

Leg Pains. Sometimes diabetes will affect one or more leg nerves, causing severe pain with cramping, typically worse at night, for several months.

Bladder Problems. When diabetes affects the nerves to the bladder, urine may be passed only once or twice a day. Between times, the bladder may overflow.

Impotence. About half of male diabetics eventually suffer impotence.

Kidney Failure. Kidney failure in diabetics can be life-threatening.

Sweating Problems. Some diabetics may tolerate heat poorly. Many develop increased sweating in the upper half of the body, with no sweating at all in the lower half. Others lose the ability to sweat altogether.

Foot Problems of Diabetics

Accelerated clogging of the arteries results in hair loss over the lower legs and feet, slowed growth of the toenails, coldness of the feet, and skin which is thin and shiny over the feet. Along with impaired arterial circulation, diabetics often develop peripheral neuropathy as well. The sensory nerves die, and the diabetic no longer feels the sensations of touch, temperature, or pain in the feet. This leads to infected foot ulcers and gangrene, which in turn may require amputation.

Foot ulcers or infections can arise from minor injuries, such as a stubbed toe, or from improper nail trimming or cracks in the skin—especially at the site of fungal infections, such as between the toes or under the toenails. They usually happen to persons over 40 who smoke, whose diabetes has been poorly controlled for at least ten years, who have other evidence of nerve damage or poor circulation, and who have foot deformities such as hammertoes or bunions.

Foot Ulcers. When superficial ulcers develop in the feet of persons with impaired arterial circulation, they are painless at first. However, they do not heal on their own once they become infected, and hospital care is usually necessary. When the circulation is especially bad, foot ulcers can become deep, and infection can spread to the underlying tissues and bone. When this happens, there is a lot of swelling and redness, and the foot is usually painful. There may be a foul odor. When infection has spread to one of the bones of the feet, the person will generally feel very weak and "ill," and may have fever and chills. A severe infection in a diabetic may result in a coma if left untreated. When the area of redness is an inch or more in diameter, that is generally a sign of a severe infection. Persons who have already had an amputation or previous foot ulcers are at especially high risk for foot ulcers.

Gangrene. Gangrene is a condition in which otherwise healthy tissue dies because not enough blood gets through to provide it with oxygen and other nutrients. In diabetics, progressive clogging of arteries and smaller blood vessels most commonly affects the feet. When the circulation is already impaired in a diabetic's foot, minor breaks in the skin can lead to ulcers which do not heal; and ulcers which do not heal tend to get infected, causing swelling which cuts off the circulation even more. Thus, infection can lead to gangrene. However, gangrene can occur "spontaneously" in a foot which has neither ulcers nor infection. This often appears as small patches of black skin on the top of the foot, especially near the big toe. Once gangrene starts, it often progresses rapidly— with visible enlargement of the black areas literally "overnight." Gangrene can become life-threatening because dead tissue provides a breeding ground for bacteria, and this causes infection to spread to the surrounding, healthy tissue. If the infection spreads to nearby bone or into the bloodstream, it becomes more difficult to treat and is particularly dangerous.

Diagnosing Diabetes

A diabetic is a person who has persistently high blood sugar levels. Merely having sugar in the urine does not by itself indicate diabetes. Diagnosing diabetes requires at least one blood test—a fasting plasma glucose or an oral glucose tolerance test. A **fasting plasma glucose** merely requires drawing a single blood sample after an overnight fast. The **oral glucose tolerance test** is a series of blood samples drawn over a three- to five-hour period after drinking a solution of sugar water. A person who undergoes the glucose tolerance test is placed on a high-carbohydrate diet for three days beforehand and must fast overnight. Persons who are about to undergo blood testing for diabetes must avoid cigarettes, caffeine, alcohol, and strenuous exercise during this period.

Although most laboratories measure the glucose concentration of *plasma,* rather than *whole blood,* doctors generally speak of a "fasting blood sugar." (The plasma is the clear part of the blood which "floats" to the top of a test tube after the blood specimen has been centrifuged.) The measurement of glucose in plasma is about 15 points higher than in whole blood. For simplicity, we shall use the term "fasting blood sugar" to mean "fasting *plasma* sugar."

The National Diabetes Data Group requires that persons who are classified as having "diabetes mellitus" be free of other conditions or diseases that might cause abnormal blood sugar levels (such as having had a fever within two weeks), and have the following:

- Classical symptoms of diabetes (frequent thirst and urination, etc.) and a clearly high blood sugar level; *or*
- A fasting blood sugar* higher than 140 on more than one occasion; *or*
- A nonelevated fasting blood sugar level, but elevated glucose levels during an oral glucose tolerance test that are more than 200 *both at two hours and at some other point between zero and two hours,* on more than one occasion.

Persons with a fasting blood sugar (or blood sugar during an oral glucose tolerance test) somewhere between normal and elevated have **impaired glucose tolerance (IGT)**. They are *not* diabetics and may not become diabetic. From 1 to 5 percent progress to diabetes each year. The following factors will determine whether persons with IGT go on to develop frank diabetes:

- Age (younger persons with an impaired glucose tolerance test will be more likely to develop diabetes); *and*
- Obesity (especially, how long one has been obese and the degree of obesity).

---

*Technically, fasting plasma glucose, as noted earlier.

The Treatment of Diabetes

Diet

The dietary management of the noninsulin-dependent diabetic is the same as for the insulin-dependent diabetic. This includes reducing calories if overweight, minimizing saturated fats and cholesterol, and increasing complex carbohydrates to 55 or 60 percent of the total dietary calories and limiting or avoiding simple carbohydrates such as sugar and honey. Vegetables and starchy food should be eaten in greater quantities, and foods containing animal fat should be limited. Increased fiber is recommended.

The timing of meals is also important. Diabetics should have both a mid-afternoon snack and a bedtime snack. Meals should be eaten promptly. The fad toward artificial sweeteners or special ("dietetic") foods is not recommended. Alcohol consumption should be moderate. Diabetics should avoid concentrated sweets. However, just how far one should go in avoiding sugar is a controversial matter. A diabetic diet is well rounded, with a proper proportion of various kinds of foods. "Exchange diets" have been developed for this purpose. They instruct one to pick and choose foods from certain lists, in order to enjoy variety. Even for diabetics on insulin, the composition of individual meals is less important than having the calories distributed evenly throughout the day. The most important difference between a diabetic's diet and a normal person's diet is the addition of snacks between meals.

Weight Reduction

The most important thing an overweight diabetic can do is lose weight. Especially for overweight people who develop adult onset diabetes, weight loss may be all that is necessary to control the disease. Even for people who need insulin, losing excess weight will reduce their insulin requirement.

Exercise

Exercise tends to reduce the level of sugar in the blood, and it tends to cause weight loss, which is helpful in overweight diabetics. Exercise will also reduce the insulin requirements of insulin-dependent diabetics.

Oral Agents

When diet and exercise alone cannot control blood sugar in mild diabetics, one of the following oral agents which are available in this country are usually prescribed: Orinase (tolbutamide), Diabinese (chlorpropamide), Dymelor (acetohexamide), Tolinase (tolazamide), Diabeta (glyburide), Micronase (glyburide), and Glucotrol (glipizide).

There are certain risks associated with the use of oral agents in older persons. Low blood sugar (discussed below) may develop slowly and lead to coma without any symptoms beforehand. One drug—chlorpropamide (Diabinese)—is especially risky in the elderly because, in addition to being metabolized slowly (reaching peak levels in about five days), it has a tendency to cause a condition known as "water intoxication," in which the body retains excessive fluid, causing a variety of side effects such as weakness and mental confusion. Other side effects of oral agents include heartburn, upset stomach, and "gas." In some persons, any alcohol ingested will cause flushing of the face and scalp and a general sick feeling, or even nausea and vomiting. For this reason, it is recommended that alcohol *not* be drunk by persons taking these drugs.

One problem, increasingly common in later years, is kidney failure; thus, drugs that are detoxified by the kidneys should be used with caution in older persons. Orinase (tolbutamide) and Tolinase (tolazamide) are perhaps the safest of the oral agents, due in part to the fact that they are inactivated either entirely (Orinase) or mostly (Tolinase) by the liver rather than by the kidneys, as in the case of Diabinese and Dymelor.

Insulin

Only a third of elderly diabetics need insulin. Diabetics who take insulin right before exercising should not inject into a muscle that will be used preferentially during that exercise. For example, persons who are about to go running should not inject into their legs. In the case of diabetics who have low vision, or who for some other reason are not able to fill their own insulin syringes, it is useful to know that insulin syringes can be prefilled and refrigerated for a week or two.

The Consequences of High Blood Sugar

Two potentially fatal crises can occur when diabetics who do not get enough insulin end up with very high blood sugars—generally over 800. (A reasonable blood sugar is below 200.) One is called **diabetic ketoacidosis with coma**. In this crisis, the body's cells turn to an energy source other than glucose, with the result that substances called ketones are produced, and the blood becomes very acidic. The ketones can be detected in the breath as a fruity odor. The other crisis is called **hyperglycemic hyperosmolar non-ketotic coma**. In this disorder, there is profound dehydration but no ketone production. More than half of older persons who suffer these complications do not survive.

The signs and symptoms of high blood sugar take place over a period of days, and are associated with frequent urination, excessive thirst, hot and dry skin, nausea, vomiting, abdominal cramps, dizziness, weakness, and constant fatigue. The most common reasons for high blood sugar are the presence of infection, stress or anxiety; changing one's diet to take in more sugar; not taking one's insulin; or an illness. The best ways for diabetics to avoid ending up with high blood sugar are to avoid eating too much—especially simple sugars; to get enough exercise; to check their blood or urine sugars regularly; and to undergo regular follow-up visits with their doctor.

The Consequences of Low Blood Sugar

Just as dangerous as letting blood sugar get too high is letting it get too low. This can result in **hypoglycemic coma**—also called **insulin shock** in those diabetics taking insulin—a condition that sometimes leads to brain damage or death. Here, the blood sugar level drops, sometimes rapidly, to about 20 (mg percent of glucose), normal being at least 60 to 70. It usually occurs when a diabetic does not eat while continuing to take the same dose of insulin or oral agent or exercises more than normal. It can also occur if the person gets too much insulin by mistake. Diabetics who stop eating because of illness should contact their doctor for advice about lowering their dose of insulin or other diabetic medication.

It is important for those who care for diabetics to understand the symptoms of low blood sugar, which tend to develop rapidly—over a period of about one-half hour to several hours. Slightly low blood sugar can cause tremors and jitteriness, sweating, and a rapid heartbeat or skipped beats. When blood sugar becomes more reduced, the person may suffer headache, confusion, blurred vision, personality changes, convulsions, loss of consciousness, or even a temporary paralysis on one side of the body. Often the symptoms of low blood sugar are mistaken for intoxication; thus it is very important for all diabetics—especially those who take insulin—to wear some sort of "medic-alert" bracelet. If severely low blood sugar is not treated immediately, heart attacks, heart rhythm disturbances, strokes, or even death can occur.

To prevent low blood sugar, it is important for diabetics to eat more if they anticipate vigorous exercise; to always carry candy or glucose tablets (available over the counter) in case symptoms develop; to be sure their insulin dose is correct; and to take in enough carbohydrates in liquid form (such as orange juice). Diabetics who exercise regularly should be consistent in the amount they exercise from day to day if they do not change the doses of their insulin or oral agent.

It has been found that the best foods for treating low blood sugar contain about 15 to 20 grams of D-glucose. Some common sources are listed in Exhibit 11–1. If none of the items listed in Exhibit 11–1 is available, just dissolving a tablespoon of sugar in at least a half glass of water will do. If there is no way to avoid delaying a meal, the diabetic should ingest about 10 grams of D-glucose per half hour of delay.

When a diabetic begins to show signs of low blood sugar, it is

Exhibit 11–1 Drinks and Foods Effective for Treatment of Low Blood Sugar

1 tablespoon of honey, jam, or jelly

$\frac{1}{2}$ cup of ice cream

$\frac{1}{3}$ cup of jello

$\frac{1}{2}$ cup of orange juice

2 caramel squares

7 Hershey Kisses

1 one-ounce Hershey chocolate bar

2 Oreo cookies

$\frac{1}{4}$ cup of sherbet

7 Vanilla Wafers

important for family members or others to treat the person promptly with candy or a sugary drink—and more than one bite or swallow. When a person is suffering from low blood sugar, too much sugar will not be harmful, whereas too little sugar may not help. If no cause is readily apparent for the symptoms (such as a missed meal), then the person should be watched carefully the next few hours. It may be necessary to provide repeat doses of sugar or candy at hourly intervals until recovery is complete.

In advanced stages of diabetes (which tend to come after 25 to 35 years of the disease), the body's nervous system may lose its ability to show the warning signs of low blood sugar. Consequently, very old persons may progress directly to a coma when their blood sugar gets too low.

In cases of persons who become so drowsy they cannot swallow, or begin to convulse or become unconscious, an ambulance will be needed. If paramedics are available in the ambulance and are informed that the patient is a diabetic, they can give a sugar solution intravenously. Persons suffering from low blood sugar generally regain consciousness within a few minutes after this measure.

When it is not clear whether a suddenly confused diabetic is suffering from low or high blood sugar, there is little risk in giving candy or a sweet drink. In cases of high blood sugar, the additional sugar will not make the person significantly worse. But the extra sugar can be lifesaving for a person on the verge of going into a coma from low blood sugar.

The Controversy over "Tight Control" of Blood Sugar

There is controversy among doctors over the issue of how tightly blood sugar should be controlled—especially in diabetics on insulin. The danger from tight control of diabetes is risking low blood sugar, with the possible consequences just discussed. For this reason, tight control of blood sugar is not a wise goal for everyone. For many, the goal of treatment should be merely to eliminate symptoms and be able to feel at one's best.

Monitoring One's Sugar

Monitoring of urine sugars is a far less reliable method of assessing control (compared to measuring blood sugars) for several reasons:

the urine level does not always correlate well with the blood level; the kidneys' threshold for spilling urine rises in older persons; urine testing does not indicate when the blood sugar level is dangerously low; and blood glucose testing is more accurate than urine testing. Many diabetics now prefer self-blood-glucose moni- toring of blood sugar.

Those on insulin who monitor their own sugars should initially check their blood or urine four times a day—before meals and at bedtime. However, after good control is achieved, many doctors feel it is sensible to reduce the frequency of checking to once a day (in the morning, before breakfast) or perhaps even less in some cases.

Testing Urine for Sugar. The following are some common ways of testing one's urine for sugar and ketones (the latter sometimes being present if one has been fasting, or if blood sugar gets extremely high). Some methods test for both sugar and ketones; others just for sugar:

- Keto-Diastix (Ames). You dip the stick in urine and wait 30 seconds, then compare the two colors on the stick with the color chart on the bottle. (Tests for sugar and ketones.)
- Test-tape (Lilly): This is the least expensive and least accurate. You dip the tape in urine and wait 60 seconds, then compare the color with the chart on the bottle. (Tests only for sugar.)
- Clinitest tablets. This is the most accurate method, but is time-consuming and somewhat difficult. You must place drops of urine in a test tube, add water, then add a Clinitest tablet and wait for a reaction. It is inconvenient for people who are not at home. (Tests only for sugar.)

Testing Blood for Sugar. Blood sugar testing is a bit more complex than testing of urine sugar. Typically, the diabetic obtains a drop of blood by pricking the fingertip and placing the blood on a chemically treated strip of paper. After a certain time interval, the blood is wiped off or in some cases blotted off. Depending on the particular test, it may be necessary to wait an additional length of time. Finally, the strip is compared against a color chart or is placed into a meter which reads the strip automatically.

About a dozen different blood glucose meters are on the market, selling for upwards of $150. There are a similar number of finger- pricking devices available, selling for about $8 to $20. At least four brands of test strips are available which can be read visually. Some strips can be read visually or inserted into a meter. Generally, strips made for a particular meter cannot be used with other meters, and sometimes not even with previous models of the same meter. Proper technique is important in getting accurate results. Some meter and strip makers provide free training through local health professionals or distributors.

A list of available blood glucose meters, finger-sticking supplies, and visually read test strips is given in the reprinted article, "Self-Testing," from a 1986 issue of *Diabetes Forecast*. It is available free from your local chapter of state or national office of the American Diabetic Association. It may be helpful to specify that the reprint is "DF 325C."

Self-blood-glucose monitoring is expensive, and not all insurance companies pay for the strips or automatic pricking devices and meters. One of its unique benefits, as mentioned, is that it can detect *low* blood sugar. (Urine testing cannot measure low blood sugar because urine only contains *excess* sugar that spills from the blood.) So patients who wonder if they have symptoms of low blood sugar can simply check their blood and know within about two minutes whether they need to have extra sugar.

Long-Term Monitoring. Long-term monitoring of diabetics by their doctors is done in most cases by a fasting blood sugar every few months. To determine how well the sugar has been controlled in recent weeks, on the average, a different blood test is done. This is the **glycosylated hemoglobin**, also known as a **hemoglobin A$_{1c}$**. Since it indicates how well blood sugar has been controlled over a longer term, it is valuable as an adjunct to a fasting blood sugar, which only reflects control at the immediate time it is drawn.

For younger persons, poor control of diabetes means having a fasting blood sugar of more than 200, a two-hour postprandial (after a meal) blood sugar of more than 235, and a glycosylated hemoglobin level of more than 10 percent. For older persons these figures rise progressively with age.

Treatment of the Complications of Diabetes

In most areas, little can be done in the way of treatment once the damage has been done. However, this is not true for many eye problems, leg pains, and feet problems. One should consult an ophthalmologist (eye specialist) for treatment of complications in the eyes.

Leg Pains. In addition to the pain, discomfort also is due to numbness and other abnormal sensations. Narcotic drugs, such as codeine, are a last resort, since they are addicting, and often have other unpleasant side effects such as causing constipation and irritability. Other drugs which have been used with unclear degrees of success (because no controlled trials have been done to prove how effective they are) include Dilantin (also called phenytoin), Elavil and Tofranil (both are antidepressants), Tegretol, and Benadryl. One of the newest and most effective drugs for the kinds of leg pains associated with diabetes is mexiletine, a relatively safe drug with few side effects.

Infected Foot Ulcers. Infected foot ulcers usually require immediate hospitalization for aggressive treatment with removal of dead tissue, intravenous antibiotics, and other measures.

Gangrene. The treatment of legs with poor circulation which develop gangrene involves a number of options. These are discussed in Chapter 18.

Other Considerations for Diabetics

Screening of Relatives. Diabetics should have their immediate relatives screened for diabetes. Some may have diabetes and not know it. In such cases, the sooner they can begin treatment, the less likely they are to suffer long-term complications later on.

Travel Advice. Diabetics should make special arrangements when traveling. Airlines can provide a diabetic diet if given a day's notice. When traveling to other states, diabetics should be sure to take enough insulin and syringes, since a prescription by a doctor in that state is often needed to obtain refills. When flying, diabetics should bring their syringes and insulin with them in a carry-on bag. (That way the supplies will be available when needed and cannot get lost if the airline misplaces one's luggage.) Diabetics should be careful changing time zones: it is important to eat meals on schedule and to make any changes in the timing of meals gradually.

Special Problems of the Lean Diabetic on Insulin. Most older diabetics tend to be overweight and do not require insulin for their management. They are able to enjoy a certain amount of "leeway" in the management of their disease without getting into trouble. However, diabetics who are lean and require insulin have no such "leeway" and are at the greatest danger for their blood sugars getting seriously out of control—either too high or too low. For such persons, it is most important for their dietary patterns to remain consistent from day to day, and to have extra meals, and extra food before exercising.

Medical Identification. As mentioned earlier, it is important for diabetics—especially those on oral agents or insulin—to wear a medic-alert bracelet or other medical identification, to assist doctors in case they are found unconscious (see Chapter 28).

Follow-up Care. All diabetics should have a complete physical, including a complete eye exam by an ophthalmologist, once a year.

Living with Diabetes

Diabetes is a serious disease that requires a lot of management. But with careful attention to diet, self-monitoring, and frequent checkups, most diabetics can lead very normal lives. Because diabetics have to be so careful about what they eat and about controlling their weight, they are often forced into following good health habits, and some may end up enjoying better health than persons who were never stimulated to change their ways. Diabetics can usually enjoy the same careers and recreational activities as other people. And when complications begin to occur, prompt medical treatment will often relieve or correct problems.

Living with diabetes is easier when the diabetic and his or her family understands the disease. Many diabetics benefit from joining diabetes support groups. Information about support groups in your area can be obtained by contacting your local hospital or local chapter of the American Diabetes Association (see Chapter 30 for the address of the national headquarters).

The magazine *Diabetes Forecast,* published by the American Diabetes Association, is printed 12 times per year. It provides practical advice to diabetics and their caregivers, and includes information about the latest scientific developments. A one-year subscription comes free with membership in the American Diabetes Association. To join, send $20 to:

American Diabetes Association
Membership Center
P. O. Box 2055
Harlan, Iowa 51593-0238

Chapter 12

CONSTIPATION AND INCONTINENCE

Constipation

Constipation—the difficult, incomplete, or infrequent passage of stools—is not itself a major condition which strikes older people. However, many senior citizens *believe* it is a major problem, and many become unnecessarily concerned when their bowels fail to move at least once a day. Many older people think a daily bowel movement is a sign of good health—and anything less is an ill omen. The truth is that it is all right—in general—if a person's bowels do not move every single day, especially in the older years. Every other day is perfectly fine, and for a few people, moving the bowels every third day, or less in some cases, is also normal. Doctors do begin to get concerned, however, if the bowels do not move by the third day, and standing orders in nursing homes are typically for treatment to begin if the patient's bowels have not moved after three days.

A change of bowel habits in either direction—toward diarrhea *or* constipation—may be a sign of colon cancer and should be brought to the doctor's attention without delay. Other signs and symptoms associated with bowel cancer are blood in the stool, unexplained weight loss, loss of appetite, and abdominal pain.

Habitual constipation is occasionally a sign of an underactive thyroid gland. Persons with such underactive thyroid glands typically suffer from an unusual sensitivity to cold weather, have dry skin, and are missing the outer third of their eyebrows. A blood test determines whether this condition exists, and it is readily correctable by taking thyroid replacement medication on a daily basis.

The common causes of constipation are failure to get proper exercise, drink enough fluids, and follow a proper diet. A diet low in fiber and high in fatty foods and sweets leads to constipation as well as foul-smelling stools.

The barium used for x-ray studies of the intestinal tract (such as a barium enema or an upper-GI series) is quite constipating. Persons who undergo such studies sometimes suffer from severe constipation immediately afterward. Doctors therefore may prescribe medication, such as milk of magnesia, after such tests. If you are prone to constipation and are about to undergo one of these barium studies, you would be wise to ask your doctor if you should take something such as milk of magnesia right afterward, *before* you get into trouble.

Once satisfied that their patient's constipation does not reflect an underlying medical condition, doctors are more willing to turn their full attention to treatment, which is usually a simple matter. In deciding how to treat constipation, it is important to make a few basic distinctions, such as whether the stool is too hard but has adequate bulk, or whether there is too little of it to cause regular movements, or whether the bowels do not move often enough. The term "constipation" is used by people to refer to a wide variety of complaints about their bowel movements—some not true problems. If the stool is well formed but not excessively hard, the movements are not uncomfortable, the person does not feel uncomfortable between movements, and the bowels move only every second day, there may be no actual "problem"—merely unrealistic expectations. On the other hand, if the stools are very hard and move only every fourth day, the person is uncomfortable between movements, and the movements are painful, then there clearly is a problem.

Changing One's Diet to Relieve Constipation

The vast majority of people with constipation will respond to a change in diet to include more fiber. A high-fiber diet includes larger amounts of fruits and vegetables, whole grain breads and cereals, and legumes (such as beans). On the other side of the coin, candy, sweets, rich desserts, and "empty calorie" foods, such as donuts and carbonated drinks, should be avoided. Animal meats, which are high in fat, should be eaten less often and in smaller quantities. In addition, wheat or oat bran can be sprinkled over breakfast cereal and other foods. (Additional dietary information can be found in Chapter 22.)

Some doctors disapprove of adding bran to the diet, preferring that one get all one's fiber through "whole foods," in a more natural fashion. Certainly, one should be cautioned that there can be a danger in "overdoing it"—especially by the injudicious use of large quantities of bran, which can lead to abdominal cramps and diarrhea. Even moderate quantities of bran can cause symptoms if one changes too rapidly to a high-fiber diet. The intestines are a delicate and complex organ which harbor a variety of bacteria that assist in digestion. A change in diet causes a change in these bacteria; and the changeover typically requires several weeks. Therefore, any significant changes in diet should take place slowly—over a three- to four-week period—rather than "overnight." Every case is different, and you should consult your doctor before undertaking a radical change in diet. Among other things, a change to a high-fiber diet, because it may be higher in purine compounds, can bring out a latent problem with gout. (Purine compounds are broken down, in the body, to uric acid; and it is uric acid which, in excessive levels in the bloodstream, can lead to gout in the joints. For more information about gout, see Chapter 10.)

Those who choose to follow a high-fiber diet should be cautioned against sprinkling too much bran on their food. It is generally safe to begin with a teaspoon of bran per day, and increase the quantity weekly by no more than a teaspoon per day. A tablespoon (or three teaspoons) of bran per day should ultimately suffice for most people, without causing side effects. One should also be warned that the abuse of bran tablets has been associated with blockage of the bowels—a dangerous condition that may require surgery.

Although all-bran cereals have far more bran than other cereals, many people find the taste unacceptable. They often compromise with a lower-bran cereal that has a more palatable taste, such as 40 percent bran flakes. Whichever cereal is chosen, the use of fruit always enlivens the otherwise bland taste. Nowadays a wide variety of bran-containing breakfast cereals are available. The bran content is listed on the sides of the boxes.

Drinking an adequate amount of fluids is also important for

keeping the bowels regular. So is getting adequate exercise. If drinking more fluids, exercising more, and changing one's diet to include more high-fiber foods fail to correct constipation, it may be time to consider the use of medication.

Using Medication to Relieve Constipation

Although most preparations for constipation are available without a prescription, few laypersons understand the differences among the various products. This can lead to wasting one's money, at best; at worst, some people may harm themselves. There are four basic classes of medicines for constipation: osmotic diuretics, stool softeners, bulk laxatives, and irritant laxatives.

Osmotic Diuretics. One of the most commonly used compounds in this class is milk of magnesia. The usual dose is one to three tablespoons. A bowel movement generally follows within several hours. Milk of magnesia should be used only occasionally. The osmotic diuretics act through the principle of "osmosis," by drawing large quantities of fluid into the intestine and "flushing out" the stool. Citrate of magnesia is a more powerful preparation that works in a similar way. It is used mainly in hospitalized patients or in outpatients who are about to have intestinal x-rays such as a barium enema. A very mild over-the-counter preparation is the glycerine rectal suppository. This is one of the most simple and gentle treatments for constipation.

Stool Softeners. If there is adequate bulk to the stool and the problem is merely one of the stool being too hard, stool softeners work nicely. The most common and safest of these compounds is known best by its abbreviation, DSS (dioctyl sodium sulfosuccinate; also termed docusate sodium). The usual doses are 100 and 250 mg. In mild cases, 100 mg a day will suffice; in severe cases, 250 mg is used twice a day. For persons who must restrict sodium, there is a similar compound, Surfak, which is sodium-free. The cost of the generic DSS may be as little as one-third that of the brand name preparation, Colace.

Bulk Laxatives. The best-known of the bulk laxatives is Metamucil. In recent years a wide variety of similar compounds have appeared on the market. They are typically mixed in a glass of water before being taken. One preparation is in the form of a wafer, which can be eaten much like one would eat a cookie. Your pharmacist can advise you best as to what is currently available. The biggest problem with these preparations is their taste and texture, which many persons find unpalatable. As with high-fiber foods, one should begin gradually, being careful not to "overdo it" until you find out how well your intestines tolerate them. Bulk laxatives are appropriate for persons who eat very little or who do not get enough fiber in their diets. Unfortunately, persons who eat very little are not likely to take in much of their fiber supplement either.

Irritant Laxatives. Prunes, the old standby for constipation, are irritant laxatives in that they act by "irritating" the intestine in order to cause a bowel movement. Medicines in this category are Ex-lax (which contains phenolphthalein—a compound you may be familiar with, as a pH indicator, if you ever took chemistry), senokot, and cascara. Cascara is such a powerful irritant that it is available by prescription only. Doctors commonly prescribe it mixed with milk of magnesia—sometimes referred to as a "black and white cocktail." Cascara is so powerful an irritant that it is not safe to use in all cases. If there is an obstruction, trying to force things past it with cascara could prove dangerous. Even the milder preparations can be dangerous when not taken as directed—especially in the elderly.

Another irritant laxative commonly used in preparing the bowel for x-ray studies—and often given in combination with citrate of magnesia—is Dulcolax. Dulcolax tablets are also available in rectal suppository form. Both forms are available without a prescription.

Other Laxatives. Other preparations for constipation are less commonly used. One is mineral oil, generally a tablespoon a day, used in the case of very hard stool—not to soften it but to help it "glide out" more smoothly. In hospitals this is commonly given as an "oil retention enema." Since mineral oil can disturb the body's absorption of vitamins A, D, E, and K, it is best to consult your doctor before using it on a regular basis.

Sometimes preoccupation with a daily bowel movement may result in the abuse of laxatives, which can destroy the tone of the bowel and lead to the "baggy bowel syndrome." Here, the muscles of the bowel wall weaken, and the bowel becomes distended with stool. This condition, which has no cure, can be a frustrating and sometimes dangerous problem.

Using Enemas to Relieve Constipation

A wide variety of enemas are available. They are quite commonly used in hospitals and nursing homes, where constipation is a frequent problem. One of the most popular for routine problems is Fleet's brand enema. For more troublesome colon impactions, various other cleansing enemas, such as tap water or soap suds, are given. Occasionally, patients get in the habit of giving themselves enemas, sometimes daily. This is not a good practice. Like daily irritant laxatives, enemas can cause the bowel to lose its normal tone. In the very elderly, the lining of the intestine can become so fragile that even the mere giving of an enema may cause perforation—a rare but serious condition that requires emergency surgery.

A Progression of Remedies to Relieve Constipation

In spite of diligent efforts at prevention, there may be times when constipation defies all ordinary measures. A common example is when one must take narcotics for pain relief, such as after a broken bone. Another example is when one must take iron tablets, which also are constipating. In such circumstances, there is a logical progression of increasingly strong remedies to which one might resort. An example of such progression is given in Exhibit 12–1. It should be emphasized that the kind of program in Exhibit 12–1 is suitable only for certain temporary situations. Problems that persist may indicate a serious underlying condition which needs investigation.

In short, laxatives and enemas can be abused. They are not always innocuous just because they are available over the counter.

Exhibit 12–1 Steps for Relieving Constipation

1. Begin with a stool softener (and continue daily).
2. If no result, use milk of magnesia.
3. If still no result, add an irritant laxative, such as senokot.
   (One way to combine steps 1 and 3 is to use Peri-Colace, a combination drug.)
4. If still no result, use a Dulcolax rectal suppository.
5. If still no result, use a Fleet's enema.

Except for occasional use, it is best to try exercise and dietary measures first. Medications and enemas should not be used routinely except on a doctor's advice. It is best to discuss your bowel problems with your doctor, to be sure they are not a sign of colon cancer, and to check whether over-the-counter preparations you wish to use are appropriate for your condition.

Incontinence

Incontinence is loss of control of the bladder or bowels. It is one of the main reasons for placing older persons in nursing homes. When older persons are living with their families, the onset of incontinence generally tests the family's tolerance level: nursing home placement is a question of how much the family can take. In board-and-care facilities, incontinence is a question of licensing. In rented apartments or hotel rooms, incontinence is a practical matter, as managers will not tolerate carpet damage.

Incontinence of the bowels and incontinence of the urine are generally unrelated problems. However, in the case of Alzheimer's disease, they have the same root cause—senility; incontinence of the urine precedes incontinence of the bowels by a few months or years. Other demented conditions and terminal states likewise cause incontinence, because the person is too weak or disoriented to get to the bathroom or use the call bell. Except for such cases, incontinence of the bowels is relatively unusual. When present, generally some underlying disorder of the intestines, such as inflammatory bowel disease, is causing the problem.

Urinary incontinence is by far more common. It occurs in older women by a ratio of 2 to 1 compared with older men. Almost half of all nursing home patients lack control of the bladder. Outside of nursing homes, about 10 percent of senior citizens suffer from some degree of urinary incontinence. Twice as many people are incontinent after age 75 as before.

Some Common Causes of Urinary Incontinence

It is useful to divide the causes of incontinence into two categories: those caused by a bladder problem and those caused by a urethral problem. (The urethra is that portion of the urinary tract which carries the urine from the bladder to the outside world.) In many cases of persistent incontinence, the cause is blockage of the bladder by an obstructed urethra. The common causes of this obstruction are prostate enlargement (in men), conditions of the urethra termed stricture or stenosis, and a condition called neurogenic bladder.

Prostate Enlargement. Incontinence in older men is frequently a sign of **prostate enlargement.** The prostate gland enlarges until it "chokes off" the urethra, and the bladder may become distended all the way to the umbilicus. The person often has a very protuberant lower abdomen that is tense, like a full balloon. When the obstruction is not yet complete, some urine can get out. When the obstruction is total, no urine can get out. In total obstruction the person quickly becomes very uncomfortable, and the lower abdomen becomes tender and painful. This condition would be fatal in a few days if it were not treated. Initially, a catheter (a tube) is inserted through the penis and into the bladder, in order to relieve the obstruction.

Sometimes it is not easy for a doctor to know, after examining a patient, just whether the bladder is really distended. In such cases, the doctor may pass a catheter into the bladder to measure how much urine remains after the patient has voided as much as possible. This quantity is called a *residual urine*. A residual urine of more than 150 to 200 cc (about a pint) is generally reason for a urologist to investigate. Persons whose bladders are obstructed not uncommonly have a residual urine of as much as 1,000 to 1,500 cc (about 2-½ quarts).

Enlargement of the prostate is either benign or caused by cancer. Cancer of the prostate becomes much more frequent as men get older (see Chapter 3). Like many cancers, it can spread to other parts of the body and can be deadly. Because it is a relatively slow-growing cancer, however, many men who have it go on to die of other causes.

Blockage of the urinary passageway from a noncancerous enlargement of the prostate gland can be managed by either surgery or a catheter. A catheter allows the urine to drain out into a bag, which can be emptied each time it gets full. In some cases, the catheter is left in permanently. A permanent catheter, however, increases the chances of infection in the urine.

Strictures and Stenosis. Aside from prostate enlargement, another common cause of bladder blockage is scar tissue which may develop in the urethra, termed **stricture**. In this case the symptoms are similar to obstruction from an enlarged prostate: the bladder becomes distended. Urinary tract blockage may often be caused by narrowing of the caliber of the urethra, termed **stenosis**. In all of these conditions, incontinence of the urine is due to the distended bladder causing such dramatic and sudden urges to void that the person loses control.

Once obstruction occurs, infection sets in sooner or later. (It is a maxim of medicine that when fluids which normally flow somewhere are blocked and begin to stagnate, they become infected.) Once infection has set in, it may cause strong, sudden urges to void, which only makes the incontinence worse.

Neurogenic Bladder. Finally, there is incontinence caused by losing the normal sensations whereby we feel the urge to urinate. This is known as **neurogenic bladder**, and often results in "overflow incontinence." (Overflow incontinence can also be caused by all of the previously discussed problems.) There is no blockage— merely a failure to know when one has to void. The urine in such cases often builds up until the bladder becomes full, and then just "dribbles out." Even if such persons had a urine container or a bedside commode at hand, it would not make any difference, since they do not feel the urge to void. There are numerous causes for this, including diabetes, strokes, and alcoholism.

Urinary Incontinence in Older Women

Women have no prostate gland to cause obstruction of the bladder neck. However, like men, they also can suffer from the other problems just mentioned—urethral stenosis, urethral stricture, and neurogenic bladder. More often, though, women tend to suffer more than men from incontinence problems of *minor* degrees as they get older due to urinary infections. When this happens they may get a sudden strong urge to void that makes them lose control before they can get to a bathroom. Women are troubled by urinary infections more than men because the female urethra is so much shorter than the male's. When older men develop urinary infections, it is usually a sign of a more serious problem—usually prostate enlargement causing an obstruction.

In older women, the single most common cause of urinary incontinence is an **unstable bladder muscle**, which contracts without the usual voluntary control. Merely changing position or coughing can trigger this instability in such women. Another form of incontinence from which women suffer far more frequently than men is **stress incontinence**. This is loss of urine upon coughing or sneezing. Such conditions are commonly left over from earlier life, after repeated childbirth has left such women with lax muscles in the pelvic and bladder areas.

In women who suffer urinary incontinence but whose bladders are not obviously distended and whose urine is not infected, a likely diagnosis may not be readily apparent without a thorough evaluation.

Treatment of Fecal Incontinence

The treatment of fecal incontinence depends on the particular cause. Inflammatory bowel disease and irritable bowel syndrome, although relatively uncommon, do cause diarrhea, and the symptomatic treatment of diarrhea, regardless of the underlying cause, can be undertaken with certain drugs. Best known for managing diarrhea is Lomotil (also available at a much lower price by its generic equivalent—diphenoxylate hydrochloride). One side effect is that it is habit-forming, being an opiate derivative. It can also cause drowsiness in older persons, which can become a serious problem during illness, when older persons often become lethargic and unable to eat. A powerful over-the-counter drug for diarrhea which is *not* habit-forming, and which is less prone to cause drowsiness, is Imodium (not yet available in a generic equivalent). Other over-the-counter drugs for diarrhea include kaopectate and Pepto-bismol. However, nothing works to stop diarrhea quickly quite like Lomotil or Imodium.

Treatment of Urinary Incontinence

The treatment of urinary incontinence is likewise related to the cause. Stress incontinence is generally treated with great success by an operation known as a **bladder lift** (technically, a Marshall-Marchetti repair). This procedure strengthens the bladder floor by tightening the muscles. Other treatments include transurethral resection of the prostate gland, removing obstruction in the urethra from stenosis or stricture, certain exercises and medications, and—when all else fails—insertion of an internal catheter.

Transurethral Resection of the Prostate. In men, obstruction caused by an enlarged prostate gland is treated with an operation known as a **TURP (transurethral resection of the prostate)**. The evaluation to determine the cause of the enlargement consists of a series of steps which often can be done as an outpatient and includes a kidney x-ray, called an IVP (intravenous pyelogram), and a look inside the bladder (cystoscopy). The treatment itself requires admission to the hospital for a stay of about five to seven days. Once the patient is under general or spinal anesthesia (general anesthesia is avoided, whenever possible, in very old persons or those in poor condition), the urologist scrapes out the *excess* prostate tissue, but most of the prostate gland remains in place. After the operation, the catheter remains for some four or five days until the urine—which is very bloody right after the operation—gradually clears. Then the catheter is removed and the patient, if able to void normally, goes home the following day.

Many people are surprised to learn that a TURP may need to be repeated in later years. This can be true whether the prostate tissue scraped out was benign *or* malignant. Benign prostatic tissue can overgrow in the future, just as it did in the past. Malignant prostate tissue, of course, is more likely to grow back quickly, since cancer cells grow faster than ordinary cells. What most lay persons do not understand is that just because an operation is done for prostate cancer, that does not mean all of the cancer is removed. In fact, prostate cancer is so difficult to cure surgically, it is unusual for the surgeon to be able to remove *all* the cancer cells during a TURP. In some cases—but not all—it is possible to perform a more extensive operation which may totally remove all of the prostate gland and all the prostate cancer. Prostate cancer, however, is one type of cancer in which a complete cure is often not possible.

Removal of Urethral Obstruction. Urinary incontinence caused by obstruction of the urethra from narrowing (stenosis) or scar tissue (stricture) can often be treated during a procedure known as cystoscopy (when the bladder is looked into) merely by inserting solid metal tubes known as "sounds," which widen the passageway by stretching it and which may break up the scar tissue, thereby removing the obstruction. Sometimes this procedure must be repeated frequently (in a matter of months or even weeks) if the condition recurs soon. In other cases, the condition seldom or never recurs.

Exercise and Medication. In the case of the most common cause of urinary incontinence in older women—instability of the bladder muscle—certain exercises and drugs are frequently helpful in stimulating the bladder muscles to "relearn" their normal function. However, in order to determine if this is the problem, a cystometrogram (a term for measurement of bladder function) is often done, usually as an outpatient procedure, to measure a variety of things, such as the quantity of urine voided, the quantity of urine remaining in the bladder after voiding, the voiding time, and whether the person can feel the sensation of a full bladder when sterile water is injected into it.

Internal Catheters. In the case of a neurogenic bladder (when the sensation of having to void has been lost), there is no "cure" for urinary incontinence. However, *improvement* may be achieved by medical or surgical means. Sometimes the person can be successfully managed with adult diapers or an external ("condom-type," for men) catheter, and nothing more may need to be done. In some cases of neurogenic bladder, periodic spasms of the bladder cause emptying. In other cases, the bladder fills to the point of overflowing, and the urine then dribbles out. Some persons with neurogenic bladder can be taken, or can take themselves, to the bathroom every three or four hours to void, even though they have no urge. Others, however, will be unable to void even if they try. When senile persons can neither take care of themselves nor tell their attendants when they have accidentally voided, the resultant wetness can lead to bedsores. (The treatment of bedsores is discussed in Chapter 21.) Once bedsores begin to develop, an internal catheter is generally inserted to keep the skin dry.

The main disadvantage of having a permanent *internal* catheter is that urinary tract infections tend to occur more readily, because bacteria can enter the bladder more easily through the catheter than through the normal (closed) urethra. This results, in many cases, in the person developing recurrent infections serious enough to require hospitalization at intervals which typically vary from several months to a couple of years. When the person is relatively young and healthy, the bacteria which cause the infection are more often treatable with medications that may be given by mouth or through a nasogastric tube (in cases of persons on tube feedings). However, patients who become very debilitated tend to get infections which do not respond to oral medications. In such cases, they must be transferred to an acute hospital for a week or so of treatment with more powerful antibiotics that can only be given intravenously.

In theory, a number of medications, if given on a daily basis, are thought to prevent the recurrence of urinary infections in persons with catheters. In practice, however, they often fail to live up to their expectations. Some commonly used drugs for this purpose are Mandelamine and trimethoprim-sulamethoxazole (Bactrim or Septra). Alternatively, or in addition, vitamin C is suggested sometimes. Persons with internal catheters must often accept the inevitability of at least low-grade infection of the urine most of the time. It is important to realize that it is not always necessary or wise to treat mild urinary infections in such persons, and doctors often reserve treatment until such patients develop fever or become so ill they begin to eat poorly.

When the urine in persons without a catheter becomes infected and causes incontinence, treatment with antibiotics will often cure the infection as well as the incontinence. Even persons who do not have a catheter can develop urinary tract infections which do not readily respond to oral antibiotics. Such infections are often an indication that there is a more serious underlying problem in the urinary tract. These cases may need further evaluation—typically by a urologist—to find out just what the root cause may be.

Chapter 13

VISION AND EYE PROBLEMS

After age 40, near vision begins to deteriorate gradually, but noticeably, in everyone. The change is called by the Latin name for "old vision": **presbyopia.** This is a loss of elasticity of the lens, which makes focusing more difficult. As a result, it becomes harder to read fine print at close distances.

Presbyopia is treated with bifocal or trifocal lenses, or with "reading glasses." The latter are used in cases in which distance vision was never a problem and only near vision is affected. Persons who previously needed eyeglasses for distance must resort to having two or more pairs of glasses—some for nearer vision, others for far distance vision—if they find bifocals or trifocals too difficult to manage. On the horizon are what might be termed "multi-focal" lenses, which have a very large number of gradations of lenses.

The major types of vision and eye problems that we will discuss here are cataracts, glaucoma, senile macular degeneration, entropion and ectropion, corneal ulcerations from not blinking, and blockage of the nasolacrimal duct.

Cataracts

A serious vision problem which strikes people over 65 is **cataracts,** a condition in which the lens of the eye becomes cloudy due to chemical changes. Patients with diabetes have a higher incidence of cataracts.

Cataracts are treated by surgery to remove the cloudy lens. In recent years, a new treatment called an **intraocular implant**—an artificial lens which replaces the diseased one—has been developed. It is now commonplace and by far the most frequent procedure used to treat cataracts. Previously, the only available choice was to have the old lens removed and afterward wear thick, "coke-bottle" lenses or contact lenses. The thick-lens glasses not only are cumbersome but limit the size of the visual field. The intraocular lens enables vision to be restored more closely to its natural state. Still, as with any operation, there are risks, and the older you are, the greater the risks. Past the age of 85 or 90, doctors tend to be hesitant about using general anesthesia for eye surgery and are more likely to perform such operations under local anesthesia, with the patient awake. Such circumstances require a person who is able to cooperate. Mental disturbances and hearing difficulties will prevent some people from being able to follow the surgeon's instructions during an eye operation, so that eye surgery under local anesthesia is not an option for everyone.

The big question in cataract surgery is when to operate. Because no operation is entirely risk-free, and because there is no substitute for the original equipment with which you were born, it is often best to wait until vision is seriously impaired before undertaking cataract surgery. If you have the surgery too early, you could well be disappointed with the results, which might even be worse than your vision *before* surgery. Of course, if you wait, you are less likely to be disappointed with the results, but in the meantime you will have to suffer. It is not an easy decision to make. It can be useful, and is often required by insurance carriers, to get a second opinion.

Glaucoma

A serious and often treatable condition is the buildup of pressure inside the eye known as **glaucoma**. The most common type of glaucoma tends to be inherited and is rare before age 40. It occurs three times more often in diabetics, more often in black than in white persons, and about six times more often in persons with a family history of glaucoma. It usually comes on gradually and without any pain. By the time such persons notice a vision problem, they may no longer be able to see objects at the edges of their visual fields. Unfortunately, the damage is irreversible. In its late stages, glaucoma so severely restricts vision that the condition is referred to as "tunnel vision." This can be dangerous when it comes to walking, where we rely on our peripheral vision to see objects not directly in front of us. Sometimes a certain type of glaucoma may come on suddenly, resulting in a very red and very painful eye. This condition can rapidly lead to blindness if left untreated.

Persons at high risk for glaucoma (over 40, black, diabetic, or with a positive family history) should be especially sure to have periodic eye examinations—preferably by an ophthalmologist (an eye specialist with a medical degree)—to detect early signs of glaucoma, such as increased pressure within the eye. (These tests are discussed in Chapter 26.) A mild increase in eye pressure may require only more frequent observation. Actual treatment of glaucoma usually includes the use of prescription eye drops—usually two to four times a day. Less often, a daily pill may be prescribed as well, or in place of the eye drops.

When medical treatments for glaucoma fail, several kinds of eye operations are possible. The most common is called a "filtering" procedure and allows fluid within the eye to bypass the obstruction so that pressure no longer builds. Persons who have had this procedure end up with a "nick" in the upper part of the iris (the pigmented part of the pupil) afterwards. This is usually not visible unless the upper eyelid is lifted. A newer procedure is the use of laser beam surgery—which can be done in the doctor's office—to accomplish the same end.

Senile Macular Degeneration

The leading cause of what is called "legal blindness" (the loss of central vision to the extent that the person's visual acuity is less than 20/200) in older persons is a disease called **senile macular degeneration**. Here, vision directly *in front* (rather than at the edges) is lost. The visual loss is in the area where one focuses (known as the "macula"), but the affected person retains *peripheral* vision, so that walking about and even crossing streets without help is not a problem. The cause of this disease—generally age-related—consists of small blood vessels encroaching on the macula beneath the surface of the retina, where they do not belong.

Eventually, scar tissue may be formed. There is no pain, only gradual loss of central vision.

Sometimes persons who have cataracts also have macular degeneration. Even with the cloudiness from the diseased lens removed, they *still* cannot read because their central vision has been destroyed. Until recently, the presence of the cataract made it difficult for eye doctors to know this beforehand, because they were not able to see the macula of the eye through the dense cataract. Now, however, instruments have been developed which are roughly able to estimate what the quality of one's vision will be after surgery.

Macular degeneration can be managed with laser beam therapy in some cases if the disease is diagnosed very early. Unfortunately, this is a relatively small proportion of people. Still, about one out of 2,000 senior citizens would stand to benefit from such treatment, and thereby be able to avoid "legal blindness." Early diagnosis requires that one have regular eye examinations.

Entropion and Ectropion

A condition that is less common but very troublesome is the turning inward (**entropion**) or outward (**ectropion**) of an eyelid. When an eyelid turns inward, one or more eyelashes may brush against the cornea, causing considerable irritation and even corneal ulceration if not treated. When an eyelid turns outward, the inner part of the lid becomes exposed. This can lead to infection of that sensitive area. Fortunately, entropion and ectropion can be corrected with a relatively simple surgical procedure.

Corneal Ulcerations from Not Blinking

In addition to entropion, there is another common threat of developing corneal ulcerations in the elderly. Terminally ill persons who become so weakened that they can no longer blink are in danger of developing ulcerations on the cornea due to dryness. In such circumstances, drops of artificial tears must be administered every few hours, to keep the surface moist. (This is but one of the many reasons why caring for a terminally ill person at home can be a most challenging task.)

Blockage of the Nasolacrimal Duct

Another common eye problem in older persons is **blockage of the nasolacrimal duct.** This duct normally drains tears down into the nose. When it becomes clogged, tears may overflow onto the face. Blockage of the nasolacrimal duct can sometimes be treated with warm moist soaks to the area. At other times the duct can be flushed out easily with an instrument. Occasionally, the obstruction is not relieved by this simple procedure, and surgical intervention may be necessary.

Chapter 14

HEARING AND EAR PROBLEMS

The most common hearing problem in later life is called **presbycusis**, a Latin term meaning "old hearing." This type of hearing loss is associated with the aging process and affects almost one in three senior citizens. Many older people try to deny that they have a hearing problem, even when their hearing loss seems obvious to family members. This is too bad, since many can benefit from hearing devices.

Most older people with poor hearing are referred to an ear specialist to make sure there is no other cause of the difficulty than "old age" hearing loss, or presbycusis. After a thorough examination by the specialist, they are given a hearing aid evaluation, which includes an audiometry exam (listening to sounds of different pitch) to determine which frequencies are affected the most. Not everyone can benefit from a hearing aid; and some people may benefit from a hearing aid in one ear, but not the other.

Hearing aids can be invaluable to the well-being of many senior citizens with poor hearing. A lot of them do not realize that the old-fashioned bulky and unsightly hearing aids of the past have been replaced with much more compact devices, some of which fit entirely within the ear canal itself! These modern devices are virtually unnoticeable and have no wires running from the ear down the neck. The fear of social embarrassment from the stigma of wearing a hearing aid is one factor which prevents many senior citizens who need hearing aids from getting them. Such persons are grateful once a concerned friend or relative coaxes them into accepting modern technology.

Hearing Loss from Earwax Build-up

In many cases, poor hearing is due in large part to wax build-up in the ear canals, called **wax plugs**. It is surprising how much a person's hearing can be diminished by this problem. However, it can be dangerous for persons to "dig it out" themselves by inserting Q-tips or other objects inside the ear canal. They risk puncturing the eardrum. It is perfectly safe to insert a finger wrapped inside a damp washcloth to clean the ears. But the cleaning of earwax beyond this is best left to a health care professional. It is not always necessary to go to an ear specialist to have earwax removed. Many primary care doctors are adept at cleaning out excessive earwax; and some will even perform this service on house calls, saving the home-bound person an expensive and troublesome trip to the doctor's office. In many cases a hardened plug of wax can be dislodged by a professional in a few seconds, resulting in immediate and dramatic improvement in hearing. In other cases the wax is so hard that it must first be softened so it can be washed out with a syringe. Generally, an over-the-counter preparation containing hydrogen peroxide (such as Debrox) is used. However, this solution can be very irritating if there are certain skin conditions inside the ear canal, and should not be used if there is a perforation of the eardrum. It is safest to consult with your doctor first before trying to treat yourself or a relative with this preparation.

Hearing Loss from Perforation of the Eardrum

In a smaller number of cases, poor hearing is caused by a perforation (a hole) in the eardrum which may have been present for many years. This condition often responds to a procedure known as a myringoplasty. It is done under local anesthesia in an operating room setting, and consists of patching the hole with a small piece of tissue graft taken from underneath the skin behind the ear. The result is usually a great improvement in hearing. Of course, if one has presbycusis in addition, this procedure alone may not be sufficient to restore hearing to a satisfactory level. In such cases, a hearing aid might be needed as well.

Acute Benign Labyrinthitis

A troublesome but temporary ear condition can cause extreme dizziness with nausea and even vomiting. You might think of it as a "head cold" in the balance center of the ear. Doctors call it **acute benign labyrinthitis**. Although not confined to senior citizens, it is more common in older people. In this condition, dizziness is brought on by a sudden change of position of the head—such as turning rapidly from side to side. Merely lying down or getting up quickly can bring on the dizziness. It is important to distinguish it from the dizziness which can happen in older persons who try to stand up too quickly, especially when first arising in the morning. This latter condition, called **postural hypotension**, results from a rapid fall in blood pressure. It, too, is more common in senior citizens, in whom it frequently causes falls (see Chapter 8).

Acute benign labyrinthitis is treated by rest, fluids, and various "motion sickness" pills. The best-known brand of these over-the-counter pills is Dramamine, but ear specialists prefer a different drug called meclizine. The main side effect of these drugs is drowsiness, but the lessening of dizziness brought about by motion sickness is often dramatic. Of course, dizziness can be caused by a number of things. When the blood pressure is normal and the doctor can find no other cause of the dizziness, meclizine is sometimes tried, because of its relative safety. However, in many cases where no readily identifiable cause of the dizziness can be found, the trouble may lie with poor circulation in the vertebral-basilar circulation—the arteries that enter the brain at the back of the neck. (The subject of dizziness is also discussed in Chapter 8.)

Sometimes acute labyrinthitis is severe enough so that the person has to be hospitalized for a few days until it goes away. This is especially true among persons who live alone and cannot take care of themselves: they would risk breaking a hip if they tried to manage on their own. Although acute benign labyrinthitis generally lasts only a few days, it can sometimes last more than two or three weeks.

Ear Noises

A common but worrisome condition is the sensation of hearing one's pulse beating near the ear. This generally happens only in quiet circumstances, such as late at night. It is usually a normal sound, caused by a small artery near the ear. However, there are some noises one might hear, such as from a clogged neck artery or a widened blood vessel in the brain, which are not normal. A physical exam by your doctor or special tests may discover whether there is anything to be concerned about.

Persistent ringing in the ears, called **tinnitus**, is often associated with hearing loss and should be evaluated by an ear specialist.

Chapter 15

DENTAL PROBLEMS

The term "dental problems" is used here in the broad sense to refer not only to the teeth themselves but to problems relating to the *lack* of teeth as well. Unfortunately, we usually do not properly appreciate our teeth until we no longer have any. Aside from the obvious benefits of having one's natural teeth—such as better appearance and convenience—people with their own teeth chew better. They tend to chew their food with five times the force as people who have dentures, and they have the ability to exert 16 times the force. People who have dentures—perhaps because of lacking this ability—tend to select foods that are easier to chew and avoid foods such as fresh fruits, fresh vegetables, and meat. In so doing, they miss the nutrients those foods contain. Thus, good teeth are an important factor in good nutrition.

Estimates are that over 60 percent of senior citizens need some form of dental treatment. The most common problems are dentures in need of repair (32 percent), cavities (18 percent), and periodontal disease (15 percent). In spite of this, 45 percent have not seen a dentist within five years. Among those without teeth the figure is 70 percent. It seems that despite having a lot of dental problems, older people often do not do anything to correct them. This is due in large part to the paucity of third-party coverage for dental work, coupled with the limited income of many senior citizens.

Major Dental Problems: Cavities and Periodontal Disease

Dental problems of senior citizens are frequently the result of poor dental hygiene. There are two general types of teeth problems:

cavities and periodontal disease. Dental **cavities** begin on the outermost part of the tooth which is covered with enamel—the crown. **Periodontal disease** affects the deeper portions—those parts of the tooth which should be covered with gums and supportive bone in the healthy state. Inflammation of the gums is **gingivitis**. Inflammation of the deeper supportive structures is **periodontitis**. Although cavities and periodontal disease are two distinct problems, there are similarities. Because of poor cleaning, dental **plaque** develops. This plaque—which contains bacteria—harbors the milieu in which harmful acid is formed. It is this acid that ultimately destroys the teeth.

Dental Cavities

The rear teeth—molars and premolars—generally are the teeth which develop the most cavities and which people lose first. They are more susceptible to cavities because of their shape, having a lot of pits and fissures. The most common location for cavities is the biting surfaces, where the lower and upper teeth come in contact with each other, and the spaces between adjacent teeth. Cavities can also develop around the edges of previous fillings. About half of all cavities of the crown of the teeth in older persons are of this type.

When dental cavities do develop, they should be treated without delay. They appear as white or dark spots on the enamel of the tooth. The treatment consists of removal of the cavity and replacement with a filling. Delaying too long may result in **pulpitis** (toothache). This is inflammation of the central portion of the tooth. In its early stages the tooth may be sensitive to abnormal temperature, particularly cold; but in later stages, if the pulp is totally destroyed, this sensitivity disappears. Severe pain, which may travel to other areas of the face and mouth, may develop. With total destruction of the pulp, the tooth will be very sensitive if tapped lightly with an object such as a pen. If the toothache is not treated, complications may occur, such as an abscess which may spread to the face. With mild swelling and no fever, it may be safe to begin antibiotics and take pain medication for a day until one can get to a dentist. However, with a fever of more than 101° F and facial swelling, one should definitely arrange to see a dentist immediately. Emergency dental referrals can usually be obtained through a hospital emergency room or your local dental society.

Periodontal Disease

Although the gums normally recede somewhat with advancing age, poor dental care accelerates this process, exposing the roots of the teeth and causing periodontal disease. Deterioration of bone support may further expose the root. This starts a vicious cycle. The exposed root is far more vulnerable than the crown to the decay caused by dental plaque. This is because the root is covered with cementum rather than enamel, and cementum has far less mineral content. Another factor which makes periodontal disease so dangerous is that it is usually *silent* until it has reached an advanced state. The end result may be loose teeth, abscesses, and loss of the teeth. Diagnosing severe periodontal disease can be simple. One only has to press on the gums and gently try to jiggle the teeth. If the teeth move, or there is discharge of blood or pus upon pressing the gums, it is important to seek dental care promptly.

One of the early signs of periodontal disease is gingivitis, or inflammation of the gums. Gingivitis can occur in varying degrees. Healthy gums are pink. Inflamed gums are bright red and tend to bleed or secrete fluid when probed. The inflammation begins in the gums between the teeth and spreads to the rest of the gums. If inflammation has not been present long, the gums appear quite swollen. However, after a long time the gums do not appear as swollen but will "pit" when pressure is applied—much like swollen ankles that "pit." Treatment of gingivitis may require several visits to the dentist over a period of about a month to have all the plaque removed with instruments.

Another factor that contributes to periodontal disease is the actual loss of teeth. When teeth are lost, a vicious cycle begins because the bone underlying a lost tooth shrinks. Since the adjacent teeth are affected by the shrinking of this bone, their roots tend to become exposed. The more teeth that are lost, the more bone is lost and the greater the chance for periodontal disease in the remaining teeth. Ninety percent of senior citizens suffer from periodontal disease at some time.

The treatment of periodontal disease is in two phases. The first phase is similar to the treatment of gingivitis and consists of cleaning the plaque from the teeth. The second phase consists of surgery on the gums and underlying bone in order to smooth out the surfaces so that they can more easily be kept clean.

Other Dental Problems

Less obvious dental problems result from physical wearing down of the teeth. When this happens as a result of contact from the other teeth, it is known as **attrition**. For example, many people unconsciously grind their teeth together (**bruxism**)—a difficult habit to change. When wearing down of the teeth occurs from other kinds of contact, it is called **abrasion**. Abrasion is primarily caused by rough brushing with hard-bristled brushes. Most of the harmful abrasion occurs on the surfaces of the teeth which are next to the gums, particularly on the more vulnerable "root" surfaces of teeth with receding gumlines.

Yet another dental problem is one that can be caused by mis-shapen (especially chipped) teeth that were never attended to. This can lead to injury inside the mouth—typically to the inner part of the upper lip by a lower front tooth—and infection of the surrounding tissue.

Persons who have abnormal heart valves may develop heart infections after dental procedures. Bacteria may be pushed into the bloodstream, where they may travel to the abnormal valve and cause a dangerous condition known as **bacterial endocarditis**. However, taking antibiotics can prevent this condition.

Persons with heart abnormalities, such as a heart murmur left over from childhood rheumatic fever, an artificial heart valve, mitral valve prolapse syndrome, certain kinds of abnormal heart valves, or holes in the heart, should take 2 grams of penicillin VK an hour before any dental procedure that may cause bleeding gums or before any dental surgery. This dose should be followed by an additional 1 gram six hours after the procedure. Those who are allergic to penicillin should take 1 gram of erythromycin an hour before and 500 mg six hours afterward. However, higher-risk patients or those with artificial heart valves may need to have stronger antibiotics, which must be given by shot or intravenously; these people should consult their doctors before undertaking any dental procedures. Persons who fail to take such precautions may become very ill with a high fever from bacterial endocarditis.

Sometimes dental problems occur after a visit to the dentist. For example, following an extraction about 5 percent of patients end up with a complication known as **dry socket**, most commonly involving extraction of the third molar. The problem comes about because the blood clot which normally forms is lost. Severe pain develops within two or three days, and there may be a foul odor. It is important to return to the dentist or oral surgeon who performed the extraction without delay for follow-up treatment.

The Importance of Dental Hygiene

In addition to dietary considerations (avoiding a diet high in sugar, which tends to cause cavities, and following instead a diet high in coarse, especially raw food, which helps to reduce cavity formation), the key to preventing dental infections and ultimate tooth loss is good oral hygiene—that is, regular brushing of the teeth and regular flossing. (Drinking fluoridated water also helps prevent cavities, but not all water supplies are fluoridated.) Proper brushing in older persons requires a soft-bristled brush and proper techniques, which can be taught by your dentist or dental hygienist.

Although 97 percent of adults brush their teeth regularly, only 35 percent floss regularly. One flossing technique requires breaking off about 1 or 2 feet of floss and wrapping most of it around one or more fingers (usually the index and/or middle fingers) of one hand like a spool, and wrapping a small part of the other end around one or more fingers of the opposite hand. The floss is then "spooled" from one hand to the other as it is used. During the flossing itself, you hold the floss tightly between the thumb of one hand and the forefinger of the opposite hand. The forefinger goes inside the mouth and the thumb stays outside. Most people make the mistake, in flossing, of "snapping" the floss against the gums. The proper technique is to slide the floss gently back and forth against the surface of one tooth like a saw. This technique will also make it easier to get the floss past a tight space next to an adjacent tooth.

The floss should curve around the edge of the tooth as you work your way down to the gum. When resistance is felt, you have gone far enough. Then you retract the floss—using the same sawing motion, if needed, to free it—and begin anew on the adjacent tooth edge or the far edge of the same tooth. Do not go directly to the adjacent tooth without first removing the floss. You should follow a systematic plan in order not to forget any teeth. A good plan is to start with the upper teeth in the center and progress backward to the right, tooth by tooth. After doing all the upper teeth on the right side, return to the center to do all the upper teeth on the left side in a similar fashion. Then do the lower teeth in the same manner. Be sure not to forget the rear teeth—especially their far sides. If your teeth are misaligned so that you cannot insert floss between them, you should consider seeing an orthodontist for the purpose of straightening the teeth. Aside from malocclusion problems which may be present (and which also should be corrected) straightening of crooked teeth is important because it makes proper flossing easier.

Bleeding of the gums is common during the first few days of flossing and ordinarily is not a cause for alarm. However, if bleeding continues more than a few days, there may be more serious disease, and you should consult your dentist. Persons who floss should be aware that, because flossing can cause bleeding from the gums, they should not floss for several days before and during the testing of the stool for microscopic blood (see stool testing in Chapter 3).

Various disorders that come with advancing years, such as arthritis and Parkinson's disease, may make it difficult for some older people to brush and floss properly. In such cases, they may need assistance. Fluoride rinse programs on a daily to weekly basis may also be needed.

Dentures

Unfortunately, because so few people bother to take care of their teeth, about half of senior citizens end up without any, and three-quarters end up wearing at least a partial denture. Even more appalling is the fact that, of those who do lose all their teeth, 6 percent never get dentures in the first place, 9 percent never use their dentures, and 5 percent use their dentures only occasionally. Another 28 percent have such significant problems with their dentures that they think they need to be re-done. Among those who do wear their dentures, 60 percent develop sores of various sorts. Some of these are caused by yeast infections; others are caused by dentures that need correction or modification.

People who do lose their teeth generally lose all of their top teeth and most of their lower ones except those in the very front. Any tooth loss should be promptly compensated for with partial or full dentures. If the dentures do not fit properly at first, the problem should be immediately corrected. Failure to use a partial plate or have a prosthetic tooth after an extraction often results in the remaining teeth becoming crooked.

Aside from the fact that dentures are not as good for chewing as one's original teeth, many people just cannot use dentures. In some people, the mouth has an unusual shape, such that the ridges are too flat, or too sharp, or the upper ridges do not oppose the lower ridges properly. Even with well-shaped ridges, many older people do not adapt to dentures and end up not using them.

Even in those who do use their dentures, there are often problems. One problem is that the bone underlying the dentures tends to "shrink" over the years (see Chapter 9 on osteoporosis). Studies have shown that over a 25-year period, denture wearers lose an average of 2.5 to 10 mm of height to their alveolar ridges, depending on the location (the lower ridge losing more height than the upper). Once such bone loss has taken place, the face not only looks much different, but the old dentures no longer fit. In many cases, there is so little bone left that it is hard to make a new denture that will stay put.

The most common problems with dentures are looseness and pain. The pain may be from an ulceration or from inflammation due to bacteria or yeast. Quite commonly such problems are caused by the person not removing the dentures at night. However, dentures sometimes need to be adjusted or re-made. Many older people have not seen their dentist in years and should be encouraged to return. Even so, it may be that an uncomfortable set of dentures is the best the dentist can provide under some circumstances. In conclusion, it is usually best to do everything one can to preserve one's original teeth. To this end, **adults who still have teeth should have dental checkups twice a year; annually is sufficient for most persons who no longer have teeth.**

Chapter 16

PARKINSON'S DISEASE

Most people think of **Parkinson's disease** as causing only tremors of the hand or the head. In fact, Parkinson's affects the entire body in many ways. Although the tremors may seem the most obvious part of the disease, Parkinson's may cause stiffness, speech problems, swelling of the feet, weight loss, depression, drooling, senility, and constipation. It may cause difficulties with balance, walking and moving, swallowing, breathing, and keeping the eyelids open. And it may bring about trouble with sleeping, dizziness when standing up, and problems with urination. Parkinson's disease strikes mostly in later life, occurring more often with advancing age. Two percent of the population eventually become afflicted with this serious disease.

What Is Known About Parkinson's Disease

Although the exact cause of Parkinson's disease is not clear, much is known about why it causes difficulties for the people who are afflicted with it. There is a deficiency of at least two chemicals in the brain, especially in certain locations where there is a loss of nerve cells. Discovery of this deficiency has led to considerable success in treatment, by using drugs that replace the missing chemicals. However, much remains that we do not understand. Perhaps this is why the drugs do not always work as well as expected.

In most cases, Parkinson's seems to result from the natural death of certain brain cells with advancing age. The current view is that something in the environment may slowly bring about the disease. It does seem as if the disease is *not* inherited. Many persons developed Parkinson's disease during an epidemic of sleeping sickness (a viral infection of the brain) that occurred between 1918 and 1932.

The Major Symptoms of Parkinson's Disease

The major symptoms of Parkinson's disease are tremor, balance problems, muscle stiffness, slowness in moving, and speech and swallowing problems.

Tremors

Although not always present, tremors are usually the main manifestation of Parkinson's disease. They most often affect the hands, but they can affect the head and feet as well. Every case is different. Some persons have head tremors but not hand tremors; others have tremors of the hand but not of the head. The hand tremor is generally worse when the hands are resting and may disappear with use. However, in some persons the opposite is true: the tremor becomes worse when the hands are moving. The classical "resting" tremor is described as "pill-rolling"—the person seems to be holding an imaginary pill between the thumb and forefinger, rolling it back and forth like the nervous captain with his steel ball bearings in *The Caine Mutiny*.

The tremors can be more pronounced on one side of the body than the other. Sometimes it is easy to confuse the hand tremor of Parkinson's with the lack of coordination of one hand experienced by people who have suffered a mild stroke. A stroke-caused tremor can mimic the tremor of Parkinson's as the person tries to hold a fork or bring a cup of liquid to the lips. One difference between a stroke and Parkinson's is that a stroke typically affects only *one* side of the body, whereas Parkinson's affects *both* sides. Too, a stroke appears suddenly, whereas Parkinson's comes on gradually, over a period of months or years.

Balance Problems

Sometimes loss of balance is the first sign of Parkinson's disease, even before any tremors appear. Difficulty in keeping one's balance can result in falls and therefore can cause serious injuries, such as broken hips (see Chapter 8). Often, the person begins to show a tendency to fall backwards. The use of a walker may stabilize the person's gait in some cases, but not always. Sometimes a person may already be using a walker when this tendency is noticed. Such people can no longer be left unsupervised, and if the family is unable to provide adequate supervision, placement in a nursing facility is necessary.

Muscle Stiffness

Stiffness of the muscles, especially in the face, is another characteristic of Parkinson's. The person appears to be wearing a "mask," because the facial muscles do not change with mood or feeling the way they should. Stiffness in the arms can be evidenced by trying to move the person's arm at the elbow; there is a resistance which gives way momentarily at intervals, so that the joint seems to move like a cogwheel. Stiffness in the neck and back muscles gradually produces a stooped-over posture and rounded shoulders. Stiffness in the leg muscles robs the body of the normal massage action on the blood vessels there. Without such motion, fluid tends to accumulate and cause swelling of the ankles and feet. Swelling is worse after prolonged standing and later in the day, but it can be reduced by elevating the legs.

Slowness in Moving

A striking feature of Parkinson's disease is the extreme slowness with which such patients move. They tend to walk with small, shuffling steps, with the feet hardly leaving the ground. The natural arm swing is reduced. A person may need help to start moving, and, once moving, the person may also need help to come to a halt. The way Parkinson's patients walk has been compared to a moving car that has no brakes.

Speech and Swallowing Problems

Speech and swallowing problems can be especially frustrating for people with Parkinson's disease. They tend to occur later on in the course of the disease. Parkinson's patients tend to speak more softly, and in a monotone. At the ends of sentences, there is a tendency for the voice to trail off and for the words to run together.

Difficulty in swallowing may cause drooling. This symptom is first noticed at night when the person is lying down, because of the loss of assistance from gravity. However, drooling eventually may occur during the day as well. When swallowing difficulties become severe, food may get stuck in the throat, and even end up "going down the wrong way"—into the lungs, where it may cause aspiration pneumonia (see Chapter 20).

Other Problems with Parkinson's Disease

Dizziness. Dizziness upon standing results from an excessive drop in blood pressure. Why this happens to Parkinson's patients is not clear. However, some of the drugs which treat the disease can cause this symptom. Dizziness, of course, increases the likelihood of falling and therefore of injuries such as hip fractures.

Urinary Difficulties. Problems with urination come about because the bladder muscles suffer from the same kind of rigidity and movement problems as muscles in the rest of the body. The person may have a frequent urge to urinate, have difficulty starting urination promptly, be unable to fully empty the bladder, and suffer from dribbling afterward. Some of the drugs used to treat Parkinson's may have side effects which cause similar problems.

Eyelid Movement Problems. Difficulty opening the eyelids and keeping them open is called **blepharospasm**. While an uncommon problem in Parkinson's disease, it does in rare cases affect some persons so much that they cannot open their eyes at all. Although anti-Parkinson drugs also help with this problem, sometimes surgery may be necessary to cut nerve fibers in the face that affect eyelid closing.

Shortness of Breath. Some Parkinson's patients experience shortness of breath, or unusual grunting respirations during mild exertion. This is thought to result from mechanical problems with the chest muscles and diaphragm, which can become rigid and slow moving, just like the other muscle groups which Parkinson's more typically affects. Sometimes the drugs used to treat Parkinson's can cause breathing difficulties. When this happens, the breathing gets better when the dose is reduced.

Depression. A large percentage of Parkinson's patients—perhaps as many as half—experience depression. Sometimes the depression gets so severe that its effects overshadow other problems. This depression often seems to be more than just a reaction to the various problems the disease causes. One theory is that the same missing chemicals in the brain that cause the disease also cause the depression. In any case, it may be necessary to treat Parkinson's patients with antidepressant drugs (see Chapter 7). When the depression is treated, the other problems of Parkinson's disease often improve dramatically.

Sleeping Problems. Parkinson's patients commonly have difficulty sleeping, both falling asleep and remaining asleep. They tend to have uncontrollable jerking movements while asleep and may suffer from vivid dreams. In some cases, the sleeping difficulties are related to the depression which Parkinson's can cause. The drugs used to treat Parkinson's also can have side effects which may cause similar problems—particularly vivid dreams and jerking movements. Because many sleeping pills can make depression worse, they should not be used by Parkinson's patients who are depressed.

Senility. For some unknown reason, many Parkinson's patients—mostly older persons—become senile. They have difficulties with memory and thinking and sometimes become confused. Their senility may resemble that of Alzheimer's disease. Some of the medications used to treat Parkinson's disease can themselves cause confusion and other mental changes, such as delusions, hallucinations, and paranoid ideas. In such cases, the mental problems go away when the drugs are stopped. Senility is uncommon in younger Parkinson's patients—those who develop the disease before age 70.

Confusing Parkinson's Disease with Other Conditions

Parkinson's disease can be confused with a number of other medical conditions, such as brain tumors in the area of the brain affected by Parkinson's, Huntington's chorea, Lou Gehrig's disease (amyotrophic lateral sclerosis), and multiple sclerosis. Many of these conditions are different enough from Parkinson's that a doctor can make the diagnosis from an examination or with the help of various tests, such as special photographs of the brain. In other cases, however, the similarities are so striking that true diagnosis is not possible before autopsy. One condition quite similar to Parkinson's is called **benign essential tremor.** As in Parkinson's disease, the tremor tends to come in later years and gradually gets worse. The tremor may involve the head, but it never affects the legs. However, none of the other problems of Parkinson's disease ever develops with it. Unlike Parkinson's, benign essential tremor is an inherited condition. Five percent of such persons eventually develop Parkinson's disease as well (compared with 2 percent of the general population). The treatment of benign essential tremor involves different drugs (such as Haldol) than those used to treat Parkinson's.

Managing Parkinson's Disease

Unfortunately, there is no cure for Parkinson's disease. Treatment aims only at relieving the symptoms. In fact, persons with mild symptoms may need no treatment. For more severely affected persons treatment may involve a combination of diet, exercise, medications, and other measures.

Dietary Considerations

There are no standard dietary recommendations for persons with Parkinson's disease. However, some patients have reported that their symptoms become worse with certain foods, such as spicy foods or meat or foods rich in protein. Therefore, some patients may do better on a bland and meatless diet.

For people taking drugs for Parkinson's, it has been noted that taking certain medications on an empty stomach may produce faster and better results. It is thought that protein may interfere with absorption. However, some persons may develop upset stomachs taking medications without food.

The Importance of Exercise

Regular exercise is very important for all but the most mildly afflicted Parkinson's patients. Without it, such persons may find themselves losing their ability to get about and perform their usual activities.

Exercise is most important for those who have become bed-bound, especially those who are so weak they cannot perform any exercises under their own power. Such persons are in danger of developing **contractures**—stiff limbs that become folded up, rigid, and no longer able to move.

Prevention of contractures requires daily moving of the various joints in the arms and legs. Although daily visits by a registered physical therapist are expensive and not covered by most health insurance policies, a few visits may be worthwhile to train family members or other caregivers. The therapist can give advice not only about general limbering and strengthening exercises, but also for exercises which tend to preserve walking and balancing abilities. The therapist can also give advice about ambulation aides such as canes and walkers, safety measures in the home, and various activities such as bathing and dressing. Once trained, family members or aides can continue to guide the patient through the exercises on a daily basis.

It is important that exercises be started in a gradual fashion to avoid injury. Exercising should stop at the point where fatigue sets in. Persons who fall easily may need to have their exercises in the sitting or lying position. Exercise programs are particularly important for persons who are depressed because depressed persons are more likely to lapse into inactivity, which can create a vicious cycle of further depression and inactivity. Finally, for persons who have their "ups and downs," exercise programs should be skipped on bad days.

Treatment with Medication

Parkinson's patients who are depressed may need antidepressant drugs (see Chapter 7). The doses of such drugs are often only one-fifth to one-half the usual dose for depressed persons because, in general, persons with Parkinson's disease are more sensitive to the side effects of drugs. In particular, they are more likely to experience a drop in blood pressure when they stand up, as well as mental confusion and hallucinations.

Drug treatment for Parkinson's disease varies according to the severity of the case. Persons with only mild disease can be treated with such drugs as Symmetrel, Artane, and Benadryl. For persons with more severe symptoms of the disease, the most widely used drug is Sinemet, a combination of two compounds designed to reduce side effects. Sometimes Sinemet is given in combination with Parlodel, a powerful anti-Parkinson drug that is used at all stages of severity. Using both drugs together may achieve better results at lower doses, and reduce side effects.

In many patients with severe disease, the response to the more powerful drugs begins to decline after a few years. The treatment of advanced cases is often disappointing, although a number of new drugs for Parkinson's are undergoing experimental trials.

Other Measures for Coping with Parkinson's

Aiding Speech Difficulties. Parkinson's patients in whom speech difficulties are pronounced may benefit from certain measures. They should take a breath before they speak and take frequent pauses. They need to exaggerate their pronunciation, and use short phrases. They should face the person to whom they are speaking. It may be helpful for them to pretend that the other person is in the next room and in need of being shouted at. They may need to spell out words that cannot be understood and even write down some words on paper. A trained speech pathologist may be able to devise an individual program of speech improvement exercises. A list of approved speech pathologists in your particular area is available from:

The American Speech-Language-Hearing Association
10801 Rockville Pike
Rockville, Maryland 20852
Phone (301) 897-5700

Reducing Swallowing Difficulties. Parkinson's patients who tend to choke on their food should realize that this problem may be the result of trying to eat too quickly. They should chew their food well, taking in only small amounts at a time and not until they have finished swallowing the previous biteful. They should make a conscious effort to swallow their saliva at frequent intervals to prevent drooling.

Family members and caregivers should learn the Heimlich maneuver, which can be lifesaving in case of choking. Your doctor, or trained persons available through your local chapter of The American Red Cross, can teach you how this is done.

Controlling Tremors. Hand tremors can be reduced temporarily by holding the elbow tightly against the body while performing a task.

Tips in Dressing. Dressing and undressing can be made easier for Parkinson's patients by starting with the stiffer side. Instead of standing, the person should sit while getting dressed. Clothes should be chosen which have elastic waistbands and velcro fasteners instead of belts, buttons, and zippers. Clothing should close down the front rather than the back; best of all are pullovers, which do not require any fastenings. Slip-on shoes such as loafers or slippers are preferable to tie shoes. Caregivers can assist by laying out clothes beforehand.

Tips in Walking. Since gait in Parkinson's patients tends to consist of a stooped posture, a narrow stance with small, shuffling steps, and the foot pointed downward, the Parkinson's patient should try to do the opposite. Feet should be kept more widely apart—about 8 inches. A deliberate effort should be made to hold the head high and keep the back straight. The feet should be lifted high, as if marching. An attempt should be made to take large steps, with pains taken to set down the heel first.

Support Groups. Parkinson's patients often find support groups helpful. These groups, which consist of patients, family members, caregivers, and friends, typically meet on a monthly basis in hospitals or schools. Participants discuss problems in a way that can supplement the advice given by doctors in their offices. Often, doctors with special expertise speak to such groups about the latest developments in drugs and techniques for managing the disease. The emotional support of knowing that someone else is going through the same problems of trying to cope with Parkinson's disease is of great benefit to many patients.

Further Information. A number of useful handbooks are available from the American Parkinson Disease Association (APDA). Some of these are listed in Chapter 31. The address and phone number of the APDA is:

American Parkinson Disease Association
116 John St.
New York, N.Y. 10038
Phone (800) 223-APDA; in New York State, (800) 732-9550

Chapter 17

STOMACH ULCERS

The term "stomach" is used here in the broad sense, as is the term "ulcers." Technically, this chapter deals with what doctors call **acid peptic disease**. This includes mild degrees of stomach upset, without actual ulcers, as well as irritation—with or without actual ulcers—of the duodenum. (The duodenum is the first portion of the small intestine, through which food passes after leaving the stomach.) In brief, we are also talking about the problems most people have when they complain of an "upset stomach."

Most "upset stomach" symptoms actually arise from irritation in the first few inches of the duodenum. Ulcers—holes that begin to burrow through the intestinal lining—occur three to four times more often in this area than in the stomach itself. Although men suffer from ulcers in the stomach and duodenum two to three times more often than women, women predominate when it comes to symptoms without any actual ulcer ever being found. Whereas men suffer from ulcers most often between the ages of 45 to 65, women get their ulcers more after age 55. About 10 percent of the population suffers from ulcers. Far more suffer from lesser symptoms of "upset stomach." Who, indeed, has not had an "upset stomach" from time to time?

The Symptoms of Ulcers

It is important to understand the symptoms of ulcers, as this knowledge might someday save your life or the life of someone you know. Typically, pain from an ulcer is located in the "pit of the stomach"—that is, in the middle of the upper abdomen. However, it may occur somewhat lower—closer to the umbilicus. It is often a deep, aching type of pain; or it may be a boring sensation, or a burning or cramping feeling. It may even be only a sensation of hunger an hour or two after eating. The pain is usually worse after drinking coffee or alcohol and is typically relieved by food or antacids within 10 to 15 minutes.

About half of patients with ulcers do not have these exact symptoms, and some do not have any symptoms at all until the ulcer perforates, or causes vomiting or the passing of blood. In such cases, there may then be pain in the back or even in the shoulder. Vomited blood is black rather than bright red. The character of vomited blood is often described as being like "coffee grounds." It is very often the sign of a serious problem. Blood that passes through the stool is almost always dark as well, although in unusually serious cases—with massive bleeding where the blood passes through before it can change color—it can be bright red. Aside from such massive bleeding, significant serious bleeding from the stomach or duodenal area will cause the stools to turn pitch black. However, black stools can also be caused by iron tablets, certain medications (such as Pepto-bismol), and certain foods. When the amount of bleeding is too small to show up as visibly black stools, it can quickly be detected with a chemical test that takes only a few seconds to perform. Sometimes the bleeding is intermittent, so that the test for blood in the stool can be negative one day but positive a few days later. Older persons who are quite stoic may have no symptoms until they go into shock after an ulcer has penetrated through to the abdominal cavity.

Diagnosing an Ulcer

If your doctor suspects an ulcer, you will most likely be asked to undergo an x-ray called an **Upper-GI series**. This involves fasting overnight and then swallowing a pink chalky liquid which contains barium, while x-rays are taken of your esophagus, stomach, and duodenum. In addition to, or instead of, this x-ray (especially when there appears to be more serious bleeding), a doctor may look down your esophagus and into the stomach and duodenal area with a lighted tube. While the end of the tube is in the stomach, the doctor may take a sample (a biopsy) of an abnormal-looking area if it seems suspicious for cancer. Occasionally, stomach ulcers are caused by cancer. Unfortunately, it is almost always too late for a cure by the time stomach cancer is discovered.

What Causes Ulcers?

Although it is not always entirely clear just what causes ulcers, there is a familial trend in more than half the cases. Other factors include stress, diet (especially caffeine), smoking, alcohol, aspirin, cortisone, reserpine, and other medications—particularly anti-inflammatory drugs for arthritis. Aspirin is one of the worst offenders and is more often associated with ulcers in the stomach rather than the duodenum. Many people with stomach conditions like those just described unwittingly ingest aspirin because they are unaware that many over-the-counter products not specifically called "aspirin" do, nevertheless, *contain* aspirin. Exhibit 17–1 contains a list of some common, over-the-counter products that contain aspirin.

The basic cause of "stomach" problems is too much acid. Acid is produced not just by the stomach, but also by the liver, which generates bile acids. Problems can occur when there is too much acid, whether in the stomach itself, or passed out from the stomach into the duodenum, or regurgitated back from the duodenum into the stomach.

Exhibit 17–1   Some Over-the-Counter Products That Contain Aspirin

Alka-Seltzer	Arthritis Strength Bufferin Tablets
Anacin Caplets and Tablets	Extra-Strength Bufferin Tablets
Maximum Strength Anacin Tablets	Ecotrin Tablets and Capsules
Arthritis Pain Formula Tablets and Caplets	Excedrin Extra-Strength Tablets and Caplets
Ascriptin Tablets	Extra Strength Ascriptin Tablets
Ascriptin A/D Tablets	4-Way Cold Tablets
BC Powder	Maximum Strength Midol for Pain of Cramps
Bufferin Tablets	Midol Original Formula

Treatment for Ulcers

Treatment for ulcers is based on reducing the amount of acid produced, or neutralizing the acid once it has been produced, or protecting the lining of the stomach from the acid. The treatment is often similar for cases of simple upset stomach, stomach ulcers, or duodenal ulcers. The difference is more a matter of intensity and length of treatment. One exception is the so-called "antispasmotics" (such as Donnatal); they may actually make stomach (gastric) ulcers worse, by delaying the emptying of food, or by allowing regurgitation of bile up into the stomach. This class of drugs tends to cause a dry mouth and may produce urinary retention and (rarely) acute glaucoma attacks in susceptible people (those who have a certain type of glaucoma).

The traditional approach to treating an ulcer was to change to a bland diet. Now many doctors believe that diet plays only a small role, and that persons with ulcers can eat anything they are able to tolerate. Still, caffeine, xanthines (tea), alcohol, and cocoa (including chocolates) are best eliminated. Caffeine is found not just in coffee but in many soft drinks as well, such as Pepsi and Coke (unless specifically labeled "caffeine-free"). "Uncolas" such as Sprite and Seven-Up do not have caffeine. Decaffeinated coffees (such as Sanka) are acceptable substitutes. Milk used to be considered beneficial. Now, however, researchers believe that milk and other calcium-containing products (such as Tums, Rolaids, Camalox, and sodium bicarbonate) often cause acid rebound, even though they may give relief of symptoms initially. Therefore, they are to be avoided. Persons who had ulcers before doctors changed their views often used to ingest large quantities of milk and baking soda (sodium bicarbonate/Alka Selzer). The result was the occasional complication called the **milk-alkali syndrome**. Persons with this syndrome were at risk of developing nausea, vomiting, weakness, loss of appetite, thirst, and frequent urination. If they persisted for long periods in their milk-alkali habit, they were also in danger of developing kidney stones, aching muscles, and even mental changes.

The most common drugs used for ulcers and stomach upset are the antacids. Because the tablet forms of antacids contain much smaller amounts of the active ingredients, the liquid forms are recommended for persons with actual ulcers. Typically, two tablespoons should be taken one-half to one hour after meals and again two-and-a-half to three hours after each meal, as well as at bedtime—a total of seven times per day. In addition, another two tablespoons may be taken every four hours throughout the night if one awakens with symptoms. Exhibit 17–2 lists the acid neutralizing power and the active ingredients of a number of popular antacids as a percentage compared with Maalox TC (Therapeutic Concentrate).

Antacids are compounds of magnesium, aluminum, or calcium. The compounds containing calcium—Titralac and Camalox—have the disadvantage that calcium can cause acid rebound. The remaining compounds contain magnesium or aluminum or both. Magnesium compounds have the best buffering power; but they have the disadvantage that they tend to cause diarrhea (just as milk of magnesia tends to cause diarrhea via its intended use as a laxative).

Exhibit 17–2   Acid-Neutralizing Power of Antacids vs. Maalox TC

Compound	Relative Neutralizing Power (%)	Active Ingredients
Maalox TC	100	Aluminum and magnesium hydroxide
Mylanta II	90	Aluminum and magnesium hydroxide, simethicone
Gelusil II	85	Aluminum and magnesium hydroxide, simethicone
Titralac	67	Calcium carbonate, glycine
Camalox	64	Aluminum and magnesium hydroxide, calcium carbonate
Gelusil-M	53	Aluminum and magnesium hydroxide, simethicone
Maalox	48	Aluminum and magnesium hydroxide
Maalox Plus	48	Aluminum and magnesium hydroxide, simethicone
Riopan	48	Hydrated magnesium aluminate
Riopan Plus	48	Hydrated magnesium aluminate, simethicone
Mylanta	45	Aluminum and magnesium hydroxide, simethicone
Gelusil	42	Aluminum and magnesium hydroxide, simethicone
ALternaGEL	42	Aluminum hydroxide
Amphogel	23	Aluminum hydroxide

The purely aluminum compounds ALternaGEL and Amphogel, in contrast, tend to cause constipation. As a result, most antacids are combinations of magnesium- and aluminum-containing compounds. As you can see from Exhibit 17–2, the purely aluminum-containing compounds have much less buffering power. One way to balance out the loosening and tightening effects of the various compounds is to alternate antacids from dose to dose. For example, one could take Mylanta II after breakfast, Amphogel after lunch, Mylanta II after dinner, and Amphogel at bedtime.

Unfortunately, antacids do not taste all that good, and it is difficult for most patients to take any drug faithfully seven or more times a day. In fact, it has been found that most ulcer patients only take their antacids about 30 to 45 percent as often as prescribed.

Until the advent of Zantac, Tagamet was the only drug which dramatically limited acid production by the stomach. Zantac does not have the occasional side effect which Tagamet has of causing mental confusion, which can be more of a problem in older persons—especially those about to undergo surgery.

A common drug regimen for ulcer patients is the combination of taking Zantac twice a day, plus antacids. Zantac unfortunately is one of the most expensive drugs there is. After the initial phase of the ulcer, Zantac is sometimes prescribed only at bedtime, instead of twice daily, at the "double dose" of 300 mg.

Another powerful drug used in ulcer patients is Carafate. It works by coating the stomach. It is given four times a day—before meals and at bedtime. It can be given in addition to Zantac and/or antacids. It, too, is quite expensive. It may be a better drug for older persons, who often tend to produce less stomach acid than younger persons.

The most recent drug to become available for ulcer patients is Pepcid. Usually taken only at nighttime (though it can also be taken twice a day), it works in a way similar to Zantac.

Deciding which is the most powerful drug among the so-called "H_2-blockers" (Tagamet, Zantac, and Pepcid)—drugs that tend to block the stomach's production of hydrochloric acid—is debatable. In general, there is not a great deal of difference among them. It may be a matter of trial and error to find which drug works best for a particular patient. In fact, there is no strong evidence that H_2-blockers, antacids, or Carafate are superior one to the other.

Although antispasmotic drugs, such as Donnatal, are thought by some doctors not to be appropriate for cases of stomach (gastric) ulcers, other doctors disagree. Antispasmotics may be useful for duodenal ulcers—particularly when taken at bedtime—in addition to Zantac. Antispasmotics may also be useful in cases of mild indigestion. They are typically taken before meals and at bedtime. After persons with duodenal ulcers are cured of the actual ulcers, antispasmotics—with or without antacids—are sometimes useful in preventing recurrence. In more severe cases, it may be necessary to stay on Zantac or similar "H_2-blockers" for longer periods—even indefinitely.

There are occasionally intractable or recurrent cases where surgery is needed. Different operations utilize different means of reducing acid in the stomach. These include cutting the vagus nerve (which stimulates stomach acid production); cutting the pyloric sphincter muscle (the muscle at the bottom of the stomach, which opens into the duodenum, thereby allowing the stomach contents to empty more readily); removing the top third or so of the stomach which produces most stomach acid; and bypassing the duodenum so that the stomach empties directly into the next portion of the small intestine, known as the jejunum. Persons who are too ill to undergo surgery sometimes have the acid-secreting cells of the stomach "disabled" by radiation treatments.

Chapter 18

LEG ULCERS

For many older persons there comes a time when they "wake up one day," as it were, to find themselves plagued with one or more ulcers about their lower legs and feet. It is important to understand the difference between the two most common types of leg ulcers, because although both are caused by poor circulation (vascular insufficiency), the treatment is very different for each. **Venous ulcers,** which are caused by poor circulation of blood *returning* to the heart, require that the leg be kept *elevated* as much as possible. **Ischemic* ulcers,** also called **arterial ulcers,** are caused by poor circulation of blood *coming from* the heart and require that the leg be kept *dependent* (dangled downward) as much as possible. Many persons do not understand this difference and think that *all* ulcers on legs that are swollen will improve if the leg is kept elevated. This only makes things worse in the case of arterial ulcers.

Venous Ulcers

Venous ulcers, the most common kind of leg ulcers, result from breakdown of the structure of the veins of the legs. These ulcers typically are on the inside of the lower leg, close to the bone that juts out at the ankle. Usually there will have been progressive swelling of the leg for a long time. Often the skin in the area becomes discolored and mottled long before the ulcer begins. In severe cases, the ulcer may become quite large, extending almost

---

*The term refers to the lack of blood reaching the tissues.

entirely around the leg, and there may be redness and tenderness around the edges.

Initial treatment of venous ulcers includes keeping the person in bed and elevating the leg. If the arterial circulation is adequate, it is also safe to use various types of compression dressings, such as an Ace bandage or elastic stockings. Sometimes custom-made support stockings, such as Jobst stockings, are used. Water pills (diuretics) are often used to reduce the swelling. The ulcers themselves are treated by removing any dead tissue, and then using various dressings to promote healing. Infection may sometimes require hospitalization so that intravenous antibiotics can be given; in other cases, antibiotics can be given by mouth at home. With ulcers that do not clear up right away, a so-called "Unna Boot" may be applied. This is a "soft cast" made of gauze that is impregnated with calamine and zinc oxide. It is changed once or twice a week. There are also new ulcer dressings such as Duoderm. When all else fails, it may be necessary to operate. A skin graft may be applied from the opposite thigh to the ulcer, to promote healing; and certain varicose veins in the affected leg may need to be tied off or removed.

Prevention of venous ulcers often involves similar measures to reduce swelling of the legs, such as water pills and elevation of the leg. Elastic stockings or bandages (such as Ace bandages) may also help. In some cases the tying off or removal of certain varicose veins (as just mentioned) may be useful. Walking is actually the best preventive measure because it pumps the blood through the veins by contraction of the leg muscles, thereby relieving much stress on the veins.

Ischemic (Arterial) Ulcers

The second most common kind of leg ulcers—arterial, or ischemic, ulcers—are caused by poor circulation in the arteries of the legs. The root cause is clogging of the arteries—something which happens in everyone to a certain degree as they get older, but especially to persons with high cholesterol levels, smokers, or (most commonly of all) diabetics. In contrast to venous ulcers, arterial ulcers tend to occur along the outside of the leg, although sometimes they may occur on the inside of the leg as well. In addition, they often occur at various places on the foot—typically on the heel or the ball of the foot, on the outside border of the foot about halfway toward the small toe, and on the inside of the foot about two-thirds of the way toward the big toe. Unlike venous ulcers, no skin discoloration occurs in advance of the ulcer. There is usually no swelling of the leg, ankle, or foot. The leg and foot are usually cool, and the skin is often shiny and pale.

With ischemic ulcers there frequently is a history of pain in the leg that occurs after walking a long distance but which subsides with rest. This kind of history may be progressive, in that the pain gradually begins to come on at shorter and shorter distances of walking, or even at rest, as the months and years progress. Pain in the leg occurring at rest is typically relieved by dangling the leg downward, rather than keeping it elevated.

Pain at rest that is no longer relieved by dangling the foot may indicate such severely clogged arteries that some sort of surgical procedure may be necessary—regardless of the presence or absence of leg ulcers. If the patient is fortunate and an x-ray of the leg arteries shows that there is only a small area of blockage, the blocked area can sometimes be bypassed via a shunting operation. Such a procedure siphons off blood from a larger artery through an artificial Dacron connecting tube to a smaller artery below the obstruction.

When the areas of blockage are so extensive that no bypass procedure can help, a **lumbar sympathectomy** may be done. In this operation an incision is made in the lower abdomen on the side of the affected leg. A bundle of special fibers called sympathetic nerves is severed just past the place where they leave the spinal cord and pass down toward the leg. Without impulses from these sympathetic nerves, the arteries in the leg tend to dilate; and this may allow adequate circulation to return. Since the cause of an arterial ulcer is poor blood flow, the improved flow then may allow the ulcer to heal. Conversely, without restored circulation, such ulcers may never heal, no matter how much attention is given in the way of local care, such as soaking, antibiotic ointments, etc.

When adequate circulation cannot be restored, there may be no choice but to amputate the foot or the leg. Just where the amputation is done depends more on the state of the circulation deep inside the leg than on the location of the ulcer. For example, a person with an ulcer on the foot might end up needing an amputation above the knee if there is extensive blockage of the arteries.

Prevention of arterial (ischemic) ulcers involves keeping the leg dependent as much as possible, rather than elevated. It can be dangerous to wear elastic stockings or to use Ace bandages on such legs. The prevention of arterial ulcers involves general measures to prevent clogging of the arteries, such as proper exercise (including walking, but not past the point where leg pain begins), a low-fat, low-cholesterol diet, weight control, no smoking, and moderation in alcohol consumption (see Chapters 22–25). Diabetics should keep their blood sugars under control. All persons with poor arterial circulation—and diabetics especially—should devote careful attention to foot care, discussed next in Chapter 19.

Chapter 19

FOOT PROBLEMS

Foot care is important for older persons because severe enough problems in this area can lead to loss of independence. In some cases podiatry care is necessary to stop deterioration that may lead to ulcers, gangrene, and amputation. **Podiatry** is the medical and surgical study of the feet, and the specialist who practices this science is called a podiatrist. Good foot care is especially important for older persons who suffer from poor circulation (i.e., vascular—especially arterial—insufficiency), nerve damage (peripheral neuropathy), and diabetes.

Common Types of Foot Problems

Vascular Insufficiency

Vascular insufficiency (poor circulation) was also discussed in Chapter 18. It can affect either the arteries or the veins, and can lead to ulcers and infection. Poor circulation of the veins can lead to pooling of fluid in the feet, known as **edema**. The backflow of the "old venous blood" stops the inflow of the "good arterial blood." As a result, ulcers which develop do not readily heal, and they become infected. Arterial insufficiency causes a cold, pale, and painful foot. Minor injuries may lead to deep, pale ulcers that do not receive enough blood to heal. Amputations are a common consequence.

161

Peripheral Neuropathy

Various conditions—most commonly alcoholism and diabetes—can lead to loss of sensation in the feet, or **peripheral neuropathy**. Such persons are unaware of injuries to their feet because they do not feel pain there. The result is that infections develop to advanced stages before the person becomes aware there is something wrong.

Diabetic Complications

Diabetics have "double trouble" when it comes to their feet. Not only do they tend to develop peripheral neuropathy, so that they have less sensation in their feet; they also are more likely to develop narrowing of the small vessels which carry blood there. The compromised circulation, together with the loss of sensation, makes the diabetic particularly at risk for developing ulcers and gangrene after only minor injuries. This subject is discussed more thoroughly in Chapter 11.

Foot Injuries Because of Vision Problems

Persons with low vision run great risk of injuring themselves when trying to trim their nails, because they cannot see properly. In diabetics and persons with impaired circulation or peripheral neuropathy, these minor injuries can have serious consequences.

Deformities of the Feet

Foot deformities become more common with increasing age. The most common deformities are **bunions**—the outward angulation of the base of the great toe—and **hammertoes**—wherein the last two bones of the toes point downward, like a hammer. These conditions not only can be painful of themselves, but also can result in additional problems because of the pressure exerted on the deformed toes from the surrounding shoe material.

Calluses, Corns, and Ingrown Toenails

Other common foot problems are calluses, corns, and ingrown toenails. **Calluses** are thickening of the skin layers caused by friction. Friction can come about in a number of ways. Excessive motion of the foot inside the shoe is one source. Another source is increased pressure on the balls of the feet, added to the normal friction that occurs with walking, typically from wearing high heel shoes. **Corns** are similar to calluses, in that they also consist of thickened skin layers, but the thickened skin is located over bony prominences. Such thickened skin is deep and has a nucleus with a deep core that penetrates almost to the bone. **Ingrown toenails** grow into the surrounding soft tissue, typically at the side margins. There, the nail edge causes undue pressure that eventually results in inflammation and infection if not corrected promptly.

Prevention and Treatment of Foot Problems

Preventive Care

Preventive care is the best care—especially when it comes to the feet. In general, the principles of good foot care apply equally well to diabetics as well as to nondiabetics. However, because the consequences for diabetics are likely to be much more serious, they risk much more than others by being less than fastidious.

Diet. Persons with high cholesterol or triglyceride levels should follow a low-fat, low-cholesterol diet (see Chapter 22) and keep their weight down to a normal level. Diabetics should try to keep their blood sugars under control.

Smoking. Those who smoke should stop entirely, immediately. For additional advice in this area, see Chapter 23.

Alcohol. Drinking should be in moderation. Alcohol consumption can interfere with attempts to follow a low-fat diet. For additional advice in this area, see Chapter 24.

Exercise. Walking is good for the circulation. However, those who suffer from intermittent claudication symptoms (pain in the buttocks, thighs, or calves after excessive walking) should stop and rest when pain begins.

Shoes. It is well worth taking the trouble to find well-fitting shoes. Diabetics especially should try to buy their shoes at stores with specially trained personnel. It is best to wear flat or low-heeled shoes, because balancing ability becomes reduced with increasing age and also because there will be a minimum of abnormal pressure. Style should take a back seat to comfort. Be sure that your shoes feel comfortable at the time you buy them: Do not expect them to "stretch out" later. Shoes should be neither too tight nor too loose. They should be made of soft leather, rather than synthetic materials, because leather adapts itself to the shape of the foot best. Alternatively, purchase shoes made by athletic footwear companies. Do not wear thongs, sandals, or open-toed shoes.

When shoes are new, they should not be worn any longer than two hours each time. Diabetics especially should own at least three pairs of shoes, and change off daily so the same shoes are never worn two days in a row. In advanced diabetics with severe peripheral nerve damage and very poor circulation, it is best to change the shoes every four to five hours.

Immediately after shoes are taken off, the feet should be inspected for redness and warmth, as well as for tenderness. If there is any, the shoes should be stretched appropriately to prevent a recurrence; if recurrences cannot be eliminated, the shoes should be discarded.

It is important to inspect both new and old shoes each time before they are worn, to be sure there are no protruding nails or ridges or other irritating surfaces, such as torn linings, as well as foreign bodies such as pebbles or even shoehorns. (It is not unheard of for advanced diabetics to slip on a shoe with a shoehorn inside and not be aware of it.)

Socks and Stockings.   Socks and stockings should fit properly, and be changed daily. Avoid stockings with seams and do not wear socks that have been mended. *Never* wear shoes without socks or stockings. Do not wear garters. *Never* walk barefoot, especially on hot surfaces, such as hot sand at the beach, or on hot cement, such as around a swimming pool. Do not even walk barefoot at home at night.

Cotton socks should be worn during the day. At night, loose-fitting woolen socks may be worn to keep the feet warm.

General Principles of Foot Care

You should inspect your feet daily, especially looking between the toes. Be on the lookout for blisters and cuts and scrapes. Use a mirror to examine the bottoms of your feet. If you have poor vision, have a family member or a podiatrist inspect your feet for you. Wash your feet daily, and dry them thoroughly afterward, paying extra attention to drying between the toes. Avoid very hot and very cold temperatures. Always test bathwater with your hand, not your foot, before stepping in. Never use heating pads or hot water bottles to warm the feet, as they may cause burns or blisters. In fact, never use any special heat source to warm the feet above room temperature, because the additional heat increases the metabolic requirements of the tissue and can lead to gangrene if the circulation is already severely compromised.

To prevent dryness, which can lead to cracking and subsequent infection, the feet should be washed every day with warm water and nonmedicated soap. After drying, they should be powdered. At night, lanolin or a similar lubricant should be applied, but care should be taken to be sure there is no excess lotion left between the toes.

Calluses may be "buffed down." One should never use a razor blade or other sharp instrument to self-treat corns and calluses. Except for the use of pads over corns, their treatment is a surgical procedure in which they are pared down and removed with sharp cutting instruments. This surgery should only be done by a podiatrist.

Nails should be cut straight across to prevent ingrown toenails. Ingrown toenails are potentially dangerous and should not be treated with over-the-counter remedies. Rather, they should receive immediate attention from a podiatrist. Older persons who are unable to care for their feet themselves should have a family member assist, or see a podiatrist regularly.

Advanced diabetics are especially advised to seek treatment by a podiatrist. Above all, over-the-counter caustic chemicals should never be used. Most salves for the feet are a combination of acid and petroleum products, and can be very injurious to the feet—especially in older persons. Moleskin and cushion pads can be used as long as they are not medicated.

Foot deformities should be treated by a podiatrist or an orthopedic specialist. Surgery may be necessary if they cause sufficient problems. As pointed out in Chapter 18, elevation of the legs is a safe treatment for swelling of the feet only if the arterial circulation is intact—something best left to the judgment of a medical doctor or podiatrist. Even if there is swelling, leg elevation will only make arterial ulcers worse or perhaps cause ulcers if the arterial circulation is poor.

Whenever you visit the doctor, make sure your feet are examined, along with the rest of you.

Chapter 20

PNEUMONIA

Some people call pneumonia "the old person's friend." This aphorism underscores the seriousness of pneumonia in an older person, for whom it is frequently a terminal event. Indeed, pneumonia is the cause of death in 14 percent of nursing home patients, and 41 percent of them have at least some pneumonia at the time of death. On the bright side, pneumonia is often curable in older persons, expecially if treatment is begun early.

The Seriousness of Pneumonia in Older Persons

Pneumonia is infection in the tiny air sacs of the lung, which causes them to collapse and become boggy with fluid; they then can no longer perform their function of transferring oxygen to the bloodstream. Pneumonia can develop from a bad chill in a person of any age. However, the person is usually in a run-down condition or sick to begin with. In older persons, an important factor is not moving. Lying motionless in bed for long periods—such as after surgery, or if one has become debilitated—is a "setup" for pneumonia. This is because the air sacs in the lung which do not fill regularly with air tend to collapse; and, once they collapse, they are more likely to become infected. For this reason, surgeons try to get patients to sit up in a chair as soon as is practical after surgery. When this is not possible, they may use other means to inflate the lungs, such as having the patient blow into a balloon or other device. Whatever the situation, an important factor in avoiding pneumonia is to become active as soon as possible and remain active. This means not just sitting up in bed or in a chair, but walking about.

Very old persons who are in failing health are also at risk for developing a kind of pneumonia seldom seen in younger persons—**aspiration pneumonia**—that is, pneumonia caused by food or regurgitated material going down the windpipe instead of the esophagus. These people, often those with advanced Alzheimer's disease, are so weakened that they just don't have the energy to marshal a good coughing response to the gag reflex. As a result, food or vomited material may enter the windpipe by mistake instead of being spit out or swallowed. Pneumonia of the aspiration type is sometimes easier to recognize because there is often a history of rapid breathing beginning in a sudden fashion just after a meal, or just after the patient had vomited.

Recognizing Pneumonia in Older Persons

Pneumonia in older persons is typically difficult to recognize; often these patients do not develop a high fever—or *any* fever—and they may not even cough. The first indication of pneumonia may be poor eating or perhaps vomiting, or mental confusion. And that may be all there is until the development of profound weakness, which is what often brings such patients to the doctor's attention.

Another clue to pneumonia is a fall in blood pressure. However, this is a fairly *late* sign—sadly, often the one that first prompts the nurse to call the doctor. Signs more easily identifiable by home caregivers are a rapid pulse and rapid respirations. You can time these by counting the number of heartbeats or breaths in a minute. A normal respiratory rate is 18 or 20 breaths per minute. Breathing faster than 30 breaths per minute is significant. It may be a clue to pneumonia or heart failure. Breathing more than 40 times per minute produces such obvious distress that most people automatically call the doctor. A normal pulse rate is from 60 to 100 beats per minute. With anxiety, the pulse can often rise to 110 or even 120. However, a pulse of more than 120 beats per minute should be of concern, as it may be a sign of pneumonia or heart failure. When respiration and pulse rate are *both* elevated, there is even more reason to call the doctor.

The pulse rate can be measured in several ways. The most curate way is to listen to the person's heartbeat with a stetho-

scope. This is often the only way to get a true count in persons with an irregular heartbeat. Without a stethoscope, the easiest way to detect the pulse is by pressing the tips of the index and middle fingers, held together, just over the inside of the wrist about 2 inches from the base of the thumb. You press firmly, and then let up slowly until you feel a rhythmic pulsation. Once you begin to feel the pulse, you keep the two fingertips in place, and time the number of beats in a minute, half a minute, 15 seconds, or 6 seconds. To get the pulse rate, you divide the time interval (measured in seconds) into 60, and multiply by the number of beats you counted. For example, if you counted 8 beats in 6 seconds, you would multiply the count of 8 beats by a factor of 10, to arrive at a pulse rate of 80 beats per minute.

When pneumonia is suspected, the doctor often orders a chest x-ray to help determine whether pneumonia actually is present. However, very early pneumonia may not always show up on an x-ray. In some metropolitan areas, medical companies will bring portable equipment into the home to take a chest x-ray. The same is true for drawing blood. Thus, it is not always necessary for older persons who become ill to be transported to the hospital for tests. Of course, many tests cannot be done in the home. And often the circumstances are such that it is not wise to delay transporting the person to a hospital, where the tests can be done with less delay. Even in cases where the doctor suspects pneumonia, the problem may turn out to be some other cause of rapid breathing, such as heart failure. When heart failure is the problem, fluid begins to collect in the lungs in certain patterns, and this can usually be seen on the chest x-ray.

Treatment of Pneumonia

The treatment of pneumonia in an older person usually requires hospitalization. A blood count will often assist the doctor in distinguishing between viral and bacterial causes. In cases of bacterial pneumonia, doctors try to get a sputum sample or at least a blood culture in order to identify the bacteria causing the infection. Bacterial pneumonia is treated with antibiotics. For the patient with aspiration pneumonia, certain bacteria are usually implicated, and the treatment usually includes high doses of penicillin or ampicillin, given intravenously. When a virus is the cause, antibiotics are of no help. Whether or not antibiotics are used, a variety of other means can help the pneumonia patient recover. Hospitals have respiratory therapy technicians who implement many of these treatments, ranging from pounding on patients' backs to having them breathe in special mists designed to re-open closed breathing passages.

Preventing Pneumonia

Certain general supportive measures—such as keeping patients warm, maintaining adequate food and fluid intake, and getting them out of bed at least two to three times a day—can help prevent pneumonia in older persons. So can annual flu shots. In older persons, pneumonia may follow on the heels of a viral flu infection. Therefore, it is prudent for older persons (except those allergic to eggs or to the flu vaccine itself) to receive a flu shot annually.

When there is a flu outbreak in the community, considerable protection can be afforded vulnerable older persons, such as nursing home residents, who have *not* had a flu shot by giving the drug amantadine (Symmetrel) once a day. It can be given until the outbreak goes away. (Amantadine is also discussed in Chapter 27.)

The most common type of pneumonia is caused by bacteria called pneumococci. Protection against about 70 percent of the strains of these bacteria is provided by the pneumococcal vaccine (Pneumovax) (see Chapter 27).

To prevent aspiration pneumonia, it is important not to feed elderly persons too rapidly. It is also important to sit them upright during feeding, and to keep them in the upright position for at least 45 minutes after meals.

An older person who begins to vomit (for whatever reason) is at high risk for aspiration pneumonia. To minimize the risk, such persons should have their trunk and head propped up at least 30 degrees, and their body partially rotated about 30 degrees to one side or the other, when lying in bed. This makes it easier for them to clear their mouth and throat of material when they do vomit.

Often, family members do not wish to take an older person to the hospital unless absolutely necessary. In the case of vomiting without abdominal pain, it often seems reasonable to caregivers to keep the person at home for a couple of days, in hopes that the vomiting will stop. The problem here is that any vomiting in older persons may cause aspiration pneumonia, especially when the person is weak to begin with. The longer the vomiting lasts, the more reason there is to bring the person to the hospital for better evaluation and treatment. Eight hours is certainly a time when one should begin to become more concerned, although there is nothing magical about that time interval. It is often difficult to know which patients will do well if left alone, and which need to be hospitalized. Further evaluation is most easily and quickly carried out in a hospital emergency room, where x-rays of the chest and abdomen, as well as certain blood tests, can be carried out and the results obtained quickly. Despite the fact that emergency room evaluations sometimes take several hours, this is still much faster than the alternative means available. In any case, emergency room personnel are trained to recognize which persons are most in need of immediate attention, so that the more seriously ill persons are seen first.

If it is decided to hospitalize an older person with vomiting, a number of things can be done to treat the vomiting and thereby reduce the risk of aspiration. The person can be kept from eating while intravenous fluids are given for a time; and a tube can be passed down through the nose to suction the stomach's contents and allow it to rest. Necessary medications, including those to control nausea and vomiting, can be given intravenously, by injection or via rectal suppository. In a home situation, doctors are often reluctant to use suppositories to relieve the symptoms of vomiting, particularly in a person with abdominal pain, when the cause of the vomiting is not clear. Treating only the symptom of vomiting may risk masking a more serious condition, such as appendicitis or a bowel obstruction.

Chapter 21

BEDSORES

The word "bedsore" is commonly used to refer to the sores, or ulcers, which tend to develop on the skin of persons who are bedbound. Technically, these kinds of sores can also occur in persons who are not bedbound. A similar kind of sore occurs on the buttocks of persons who are confined to wheelchairs. A more accurate term would be, "pressure sores," because these sores tend to occur at "pressure points." Pressure points are areas of the body where there is a bony prominence that frequently presses the overlying skin against a hard surface.

How Do You Get Bedsores?

Bedsores, or pressure sores, occur because of *prolonged pressure* on vulnerable areas of skin. This pressure is of two types: (1) direct, "compression" pressure and (2) indirect pressure, either from *friction* on the surface of the skin, or from *shearing* forces which push different layers of the skin in different directions. Often, pressure sores result from both kinds of pressure.

Sores caused by direct pressure occur because the pressure is too great, too prolonged, or both. Immobile persons who sit up in wheelchairs (or any chair, for that matter) are especially at risk for developing pressure sores on their "sitting bones"—the ischial tuberosities. That is because such locations have more weight resting on a smaller area.

Persons who lie in hospital beds (in the hospital, nursing home, or at home) with the head of the bed elevated become subject to a *shearing force* at the base of their spine (the "sacrum"). This is because that part tends to slide downward when the head of the bed is raised. A similar type of indirect force might be inflicted were such a patient washed by a caregiver who used a rough towel to dry such skin with a back-and-forth motion, causing *friction*.

Whether the pressure is direct or indirect, exposure to prolonged high pressures may take place for any number of reasons. An important factor almost always present is profound weakness, so that the person fails to move about often. Another important factor—one which makes the skin more vulnerable to such pressure—is excessive moisture, the most common cause of which is incontinence.

It should come as no surprise to learn that the elderly—particularly those who become hospitalized or move to nursing homes—tend to get bedsores the most. In fact, 70 percent of bedsores occur in persons over age 70; and 3 to 5 percent of all patients who are hospitalized develop bedsores. A way of predicting, in an objective fashion, just which persons are likely to get pressure sores was developed in the Norton Score, shown in Exhibit 21–1. Persons with a score of 14 points or less are at high risk. Persons at especially high risk are those who have suffered paralysis, become dehydrated, or are comatose.

Location of Bedsores

Ninety-five percent of bedsores occur below the waist. The most common location is the sacrum, where 40 percent are found. Twenty-five percent occur over the ischial tuberosities, and 25 percent over the greater trochanters (that part of the thigh bone which projects out from the hip socket). Somewhat less common locations are the heels and between the knees. (The knee pressure sores most often occur between the knees, from both knees being pressed against each other.) A less common area is the rib cage—typically the mid- to lower portion, in back.

Recognizing a Bedsore

An early pressure sore is defined as an area of redness that has been present more than 24 hours. After that, the sore may blister and darken in color, often turning black. As the pressure sore worsens, the outer layer of skin sloughs, and an ulcer develops.

Exhibit 21–1 The Norton Score: Predicting Persons at Risk for Developing Bedsores

General Physical Condition:		Mental State	
Good	4	Alert	4
Fair	3	Apathetic	3
Poor	2	Confused	2
Very bad	1	Stuporous	1
Activity		Mobility	
Ambulatory	4	Full	4
Needing assistance	3	Slightly limited	3
Chairbound	2	Very limited	2
Bedbound	1	Not moving	1
Incontinence			
Not incontinent	4		
Occasionally	3		
Usually urinary	2		
Bowel and bladder	1		

Some ulcers are wide and shallow; others are narrow but go very deep. Once they go sufficiently deep, some degree of infection sets in, which may give off a foul-smelling odor. The edge of an open ulcer is almost always reddened, and the redness may extend to various distances beyond the edge of the ulcer.

Not all bedsores worsen, once discovered. Some clear up. Others remain about the same for long periods. When they do deteriorate, the best description of how rapidly they can worsen is—more quickly than many people would believe. Visible deterioration literally "overnight" is not unusual.

Preventing Bedsores

Preventing bedsores involves a great deal of attention in many areas. Proper positioning, skin care, paraphernalia to reduce pressure, and proper nutrition are all important.

Positioning

A patient in bed should be turned every two hours. Bedbound persons who are at risk for pressure sores should not have the heads of their beds elevated, since that tends to produce a shearing force on the sacrum. Persons in wheelchairs or chairs should do "push-ups" for a minute or two every couple of hours if they are able. If they are unable, they should rock themselves, or be rocked, forward and back or from side to side.

Once bedsores have developed, it is important to keep the patient off the area entirely. Even a few minutes of pressure on the sore can cause further deterioration. Persons with sacral pressure sores, for example, should not be left lying flat on their backs. They can be positioned instead at 30 degrees to either side. Likewise, persons who have trochanter sores (over their hip bones) can be left on their backs or positioned at 30 degrees to the other side—never, of course, being left to lie on the affected side.

In moving the patient, it is important to use "log-rolling" movements to avoid friction and shearing motions. Care should be taken not to shove or pull the patient across or up or down the bedsheets. When "log-rolling" motions cannot reposition a patient properly, the patient should be lifted completely off the surface and placed down gently at the desired location.

When a patient has ulcers between the knees, it is important to place one or more pillows between the knees. Pillows are also useful in maintaining other body positions to reduce pressure and friction on bedsores.

Skin Care

The main concern is to keep the skin clean and dry. This especially means prompt cleaning and drying of incontinent events. It may be necessary to keep a catheter—either external or internal—in place to achieve this goal. In many cases, the drawbacks of a permanent internal catheter (increased chance of urinary infections) are dwarfed by the much greater threat to life and limb from bad pressure sores. Much depends on whether the patient can promptly notify the caregiver of an incontinent event.

When the skin is washed, it should be patted dry, rather than rubbed, to avoid friction and shearing forces. In early pressure sores (manifested by only redness of the skin), A and D Ointment, applied sparingly two to three times a day, often causes dramatic improvement.

Paraphernalia for Reducing Pressure

A wide variety of paraphernalia can be used to reduce pressure over vulnerable areas, including the following:

Overhead Frame and Trapeze. This is a bar which is placed over the bed, with a triangular metal trapeze hanging from it. The patient must be alert and strong to take advantage of it. The purpose is to make it easier for a patient to move about using the arms. It is most useful in cases of persons who are only partially paralyzed.

Sheepskin. A sheepskin pad under the hips or lower back is often helpful. Likewise, sheepskin booties can help prevent heel and foot ulcers.

Foam Rubber Protectors. A variety of foam rubber devices are made which reduce pressure on the heels. Some fit around the lower legs, others directly around the heel and foot. Some of the very bulky ones are called "space boots." Similar to the heel protectors are foam rubber pads with velcro straps designed for the elbows, called "elbow protectors."

Wheelchair or Chair Pads. A variety of chair or wheelchair pads are made. The cheapest, though not the most effective, are simple foam rubber pads. The Jobst Hydro-Float Cushion is one of the best cushions for wheelchair use.

Mattresses. Egg-crate foam rubber mattresses are relatively inexpensive and often suffice. Air or water mattresses are better but more expensive. Air-fluidized beds, such as the Clinitron Bed, are best of all, although some are quite expensive and cumbersome (weighing up to 2,000 lb).

Proper Nutrition

If a person's protein stores are low (as indicated by a low serum protein or albumin level on a chemistry panel), a diet high in protein may be needed to assist the body's healing powers. If intake is deficient, it is important to provide foods that are calorie-dense, as well. Adequate caloric intake is just as important as adequate protein intake. Here, nutritional supplements such as Ensure may be helpful. Vitamin C and zinc are important to wound healing and are often prescribed by doctors for patients with bedsores. Persons who cannot eat in the normal fashion may need to be fed through artificial means, such as feeding tubes, in order to maintain proper nutrition. Such feeding tubes are passed through the nose and down into the stomach.

In addition to the measures just described, there are many others which are beyond the scope of this book. Visiting nurses have particular expertise in the prevention and treatment of bedsores, and can be very helpful to the caregiver in this area.

Treatment of Serious Bedsores

Once pressure sores have deteriorated, they generally are infected and contain dead tissue as well. Proper healing cannot take place without the removal of the dead tissue and treatment of the infection. Once this is accomplished, there are a variety of dressings which can aid the healing process.

Badly infected pressure sores usually require hospitalization for at least a week so that intravenous antibiotics can be administered. In minor cases, infection is often handled with povidone-iodine (Betadine brand) solution applied every eight hours until healing has taken place.

Dead tissue is removed either by mechanically cutting it away or by applying enzymatic preparations which "eat" it away. (The latter may suffice in less serious cases.) Once all th. dead tissue has been removed and the infection treated, a variety of surgical dressings can be applied. There is much debate as to which dressings are most effective, but there is no disagreement over their being more effective than simply letting a scab form by exposure to the air. Dressings are changed every four to eight hours.

Bedsores that deteriorate may enlarge to the size of a fist or even larger. Infection from large bedsores may spread throughout the bloodstream to the entire body, making the patient very ill. In about 40 percent of such cases the infection also spreads to the underlying bone. Infection of bone is always a serious condition. Very deep pressure sores of the hip or sacral area may tunnel through into the abdominal cavity. Ultimately, infection from the largest bedsores may cause death.

The deepest pressure sores generally require surgery. The dead tissue is removed, and the ulcer is covered over with healthy skin. Without such surgery, healing might take many, many months and result in unsatisfactory scar tissue covering the site. Such scar tissue is more likely than a skin graft to break down and cause another pressure sore. In surgery for a large ulcer, a square of skin is taken from the thigh and transplanted over the gap. In some cases nearby muscle and skin are moved over to cover the under-lying bone. When infection from a pressure sore has spread to the bones of the toes, amputation is sometimes lifesaving.

Part II

PREVENTIVE MEASURES

Chapter 22

DIET

Of all the habits that affect one's health, diet is the one where changes can most easily be made. This is because you can make choices every time you eat. Although most people associate "dieting" with self-denial, one does not have to suffer to follow a proper diet. Most people who follow the wrong diet do so out of sheer ignorance. In fact, there is no reason why a proper diet needs to be unpalatable or difficult to follow.

The main question is what sort of diet is right for you. Men—particularly those with high cholesterol levels—are inherently at higher risk for heart trouble than are women. They therefore should be more attentive to restricting cholesterol and saturated fats. Women, on the other hand, are at higher risk for osteoporosis and should be more concerned about dietary calcium. Obese persons of either sex need to restrict calories. All persons should follow certain guidelines to reduce their chances of cancer. This chapter gives advice in these and other important areas of nutrition.

All persons are advised to follow a diet which is moderately limited in fat—30 percent of calories as fat instead of the 40 percent currently eaten by the average American. This can be easily accomplished by learning to identify those foods that are especially bad for you and avoiding them entirely. Such a moderate diet is both a healthy and a realistic goal for most adults.

Diet and Cholesterol

Why All the Fuss About Cholesterol?

Excess cholesterol tends to be deposited on the walls of the arteries, where it may eventually cause clogging. This can result in

181

chest pain that occurs with exertion (angina), heart attacks, heart rhythm disturbances, strokes, leg ulcers, and gangrene of the legs and feet. During the past 15 years, research on cholesterol has produced convincing evidence that lowering one's cholesterol level can markedly reduce, or even reverse, these harmful effects.

In October 1987, the National Heart, Lung, and Blood Institute (NHLBI) became sufficiently concerned about cholesterol's effects that it published a report for doctors called *Adult Cholesterol Treatment Recommendations*. The institute's recommendations call for 65 percent of all adults to change their diets! Details of those recommendations are discussed in Chapter 2. All adults with a cholesterol level of 200 or more—particularly men who have already had a heart attack or who have any "risk factors" (listed in Chapter 2)—are advised to follow a diet designed to lower cholesterol. **Adults under age 60 who do not succeed with the moderately restricted diet are advised to advance to a more severely restricted diet in which saturated fats are limited to less than 7 percent of calories and daily cholesterol to less than 200 mg.** In other aspects, the severely restricted diet is the same as the moderately restricted diet (discussed below).

For people over 60, there is much less evidence about the benefit of following a low-cholesterol diet. Such persons are usually not advised to follow the more severely restricted diet. The NHLBI recommends that the doctor consider a diet less strict than even the moderately restricted diet in certain cases. However, the NHLBI still feels that, if the moderately restricted diet can be followed without hardship, even persons over 60 are likely to benefit just as much as younger persons. In the case of persons under 60 with high cholesterol, some may need additional treatment with drugs if the more stringent diet fails to lower cholesterol sufficiently.

The so-called Step 1 (moderately restricted) cholesterol-lowering diet recommended by the NHLBI **limits total fat to 30 percent of all calories, cholesterol to less than 300 mg per day, saturated fatty acids to less than 10 percent of total calories, polyunsaturated fatty acids to 10 percent of total calories, and recommends that monounsaturated fatty acids comprise 10 to 15 percent of total calories.** Protein should comprise 10 to 20 percent of total calories. Total calories should be limited to the amount required to achieve and maintain a desirable weight.

The Step 2 (severely restricted) diet of the NHLBI is recommended only for those persons under age 60 whose cholesterol does not come down sufficiently after 3 months of the Step 1 diet. The assistance of a registered dietician is encouraged for this more stringent diet.

The high cholesterol levels of Americans are due to a combination of factors. An important fact most people don't appreciate is that the body can make cholesterol on its own, even with no cholesterol in the diet. The most important factor is the intake of saturated fats, which is responsible for about 60 percent of excess cholesterol. The current average intake of such saturated fats is 13 to 15 percent of total calories, but many Americans consume 15 to 20 percent of their calories in this way. The next most important factor is the intake of cholesterol itself, responsible for some 25 percent of excess cholesterol. The current average intake is about 250 to 450 mg per day. Obesity is responsible for about 5 percent. However, it is hard to separate obesity from other factors. The problem is akin to the question of the chicken and the egg (which came first?), because the most common cause of high cholesterol—high intake of saturated fats—also tends to cause obesity. Finally, the lack of adequate fiber in the diet is responsible for about 5 percent of excess cholesterol. Without all these factors, the average cholesterol level of most people would be about 140 mg.

Persons whose cholesterol levels are too high should follow a low-cholesterol and low-fat diet, with the emphasis on limiting *highly saturated* fatty acids. Highly saturated fatty acids contain a high ratio of hydrogen to carbon atoms. A fatty acid that lacks only two hydrogen atoms from being fully "saturated" is said to be *monounsaturated*. Olive oil is such an example. If more than two hydrogen atoms are "missing" from the "fully saturated state," the fatty acid is *polyunsaturated*. Corn oil is such an example. Foods that contain a significant amount of saturated fats are meats and most milk products. Even though fat is more important than cholesterol in following a low-fat-and-cholesterol diet, one should be careful not to "go overboard" in the amount of cholesterol eaten. Eggs are so very high in cholesterol that the NHLBI recommends they be limited to three per week on the moderately restricted diet, and one per week on the severely restricted diet. Other foods high in cholesterol—such as beef liver and organ meats—should be severely limited.

To get a better idea of what foods to avoid, it may be useful to ponder the fact that a strict vegetarian diet (avoiding eggs, milk products, and fish, in addition to meat and fowl) is very low in fat. And, there is no cholesterol whatsoever in vegetables, cereal grains, starches, and fruits. By comparison, almost everything else tends to promote a high cholesterol level.

The Amount of Cholesterol in Common Foods

A diet high in cholesterol has more than 500 mg per day, while one low in cholesterol has less than 300 mg per day. Changing to a low-cholesterol diet means becoming knowledgeable about the amount of cholesterol in the foods most of us tend to consume each day.

Fats and Oils. Vegetable oils, margarine, and peanut butter have *no* cholesterol. A tablespoon of butter has 31 mg, lard 12 mg, and mayonnaise 8 mg. These are quite modest amounts. Thus, fats and oils contain little or no cholesterol themselves.

Baked Goods. Donuts, cookies, and frosted cake are relatively modest in cholesterol, varying from 10 to 50 mg per portion.

Milk and Dairy Products. Aside from ice cream, which contains 59 mg of cholesterol per cup, most milk products are more modest in their cholesterol content. Whole milk contains 33 mg per cup, and most cheeses, including regular cottage cheese, contain about 25 to 35 mg per cup. Low-fat (1 percent) cottage cheese contains only 10 mg per cup.

Animal Meats, Including Fowl and Fish. All these are somewhat higher in cholesterol. A 3-oz serving of most cuts of beef, including hamburger, varies from 65 to 90 mg of cholesterol. Veal, lamb, chicken, and turkey are similar. Both lean and fatty fish have around 60 mg of cholesterol per serving. Some shellfish, however, are slightly higher, and some considerably higher. Per 3½-oz serving, shrimp, crayfish, and lobster have about 90 to 150 mg. Most other shellfish contain from 35 to 85 mg per portion. Scallops, though, contain only 24 mg per portion, and mussels 28 mg. At the other extreme, calamari have 233 gm. Delicatessen-type meat products, such as hot dogs, salami, or beef bologna, contain about 15 to 45 mg of cholesterol per slice, making them comparable to regular beef products when comparing similarly sized portions. Pork products are similar to beef in their cholesterol content except for cured bacon, which has only 16 mg for 3 slices, and spareribs, which have 103 mg of cholesterol per serving. Beef liver is extremely high in cholesterol, with 372 mg per 3-oz portion. Calf, hog, and lamb liver are similar in cholesterol content. Meats that are less commonly eaten, but exceedingly high in cholesterol, are beef kidney (600 mg per 3-oz portion), sweetbreads (400 mg), and brains (1,700 mg). Chicken gizzard has 283 mg per portion.

Eggs. The yolk of one large egg contains 274 mg of cholesterol. The white contains only a trace. One can see that a breakfast with two eggs contains over 500 mg of cholesterol—a high amount for the day, even if one were to eat no cholesterol-containing foods at lunch and dinner. Those who do not wish to eliminate eggs from their diet entirely are free to eat the whites of the egg. (The whites, incidentally, contain all of the protein in the egg.) This can be done by substituting egg whites for whole eggs in recipes. In addition, one can simply discard the yolks of the eggs when they are served.

The Amount of Saturated Fats in Common Foods

As mentioned, the current recommendation calls for adults to reduce the amount of calories from fat to 30 percent. Fat has more than twice the calories per gram—9—than proteins and carbohydrates, which each have 4 calories per gram. Since most people consume 1,500 to 2,500 calories per day, this means a **limit of 50 to 83 grams of fat.** Furthermore, *saturated* fatty acids should constitute less than 10 percent of total calories. Thus, only a third of all fatty acids should be *saturated*. This is a limit of **16 to 27** grams per day of saturated fatty acids. Keeping these figures in mind, let us review various foods:

Fats and Oils. Fats and oils are mixtures, with the saturation less than 100 percent. Fats or oils are termed either *saturated, polyunsaturated* or *monounsaturated* because such fatty acids predominate in the mixture. Saturated fats tend to be solids, while polyunsaturated fats tend to be liquids, at room temperature (although there are exceptions, such as coconut oil and palm kernel oil). Saturated fats tend to be cheaper and have a longer shelf life in stores. They therefore tend to be used in products such as candy bars that are sold in vending machines or that may remain on shelves for weeks or months before being sold. The degree of saturation—and home shelf life—can be increased by a process known as *hydrogenation*. Thus, vegetable products such as corn oil margarine can end up more saturated through hydrogenation, even though they may have started out in a highly polyunsaturated state. One can check the label to find out if hydrogenation has taken place. Vegetable oils with a predominance of saturated fatty acids (here listed as a percentage of the total) are coconut oil (87 percent), palm kernel oil (80 percent), and palm oil (81 percent). Butter has 61 percent of its fat as saturated fatty acids.

Let us now consider various foods in terms of their *weight* of fat per portion. Coconut oil and palm kernel oil have the most saturated fat of any food products—12 and 11 grams per tablespoon (respectively), followed by palm oil and butter, each of which have 7 grams per tablespoon. These substances are considerably higher than peanut, corn, and olive oils, and corn oil and soybean margarines, each of which has only 2 grams of saturated fat per tablespoon. Sunflower and safflower oil and soybean oil tub margarine each have only 1 gram of saturated fat per tablespoon.

Baked goods, processed foods, popcorn oils, and nondairy creamers tend to contain highly saturated vegetable oils, such as palm kernel oil, palm oil, and coconut oil.

Meats. In general, animal meat has about half as much saturated fat as coconut oil and palm kernel oil. Pork has from 4 to 7 grams of saturated fat per 3-oz portion, depending on the cut. Pork spareribs are even worse, with 10 grams. Frankfurters have 7 grams each. Ground beef with 20 percent fat also has 7 grams per 3-oz portion. With 15 percent fat, ground beef has only 5 grams per portion, which is comparable with certain other fatty cuts of beef, such as brisket, rib roast, and short ribs. The leanest cuts of beef—top round, eye round, London broil, filet mignon, tenderloin, and sirloin tip—vary from 2 to 3 grams of saturated fat per portion. Veal and lamb are slightly higher, at 4 grams each.

The traditional categories of labeling have made the fattest meats seem the most attractive. "Prime" has the highest fat content, "good" the least, and "choice" intermediate. Most graded beef is "choice." Ungraded beef—called "select"—tends to be "good." When meat is not graded, the best clue to the amount of fat is the degree of marbling—the streaks or specks of fat seen on the inside. The leanest beef has the least marbling.

When cooking meat, there are ways to reduce the amount of fat eaten. Begin by trimming the outside fat beforehand. Broil meat so that the fat can drip off. And be sure to drain the fat when sautéing.

Fowl. Chicken and turkey are relatively low in saturated fat, especially the white meat portions. The skin should be discarded because of its high fat content.

Milk and Milk Products. Regular ice cream tops the list with 9 grams of saturated fat per 1-cup portion. This is followed by whole milk and most cheeses, which have 4 to 6 grams per cup or 1-oz portion. Low-fat 2 percent milk has 3.3 grams of saturated fat per cup; low-fat 1 percent milk, 2 grams. Low-fat cottage cheese (1 percent fat) and yogurt made with low-fat milk each have only 2 grams of saturated fat per cup.

Eggs. Eggs have no saturated fat.

Baked Goods. Frosted cakes have from 3 to 5 grams of saturated fat per piece. Cake donuts have 1 gram, and yeast donuts, 3 grams of saturated fat.

Fish. Even fatty fish has only 1 gram of saturated fat per 3-oz serving. Otherwise, fish, including shellfish, has less than ½ gram per portion. Keeping in mind that shrimp, lobster, and especially calamari tend to be rather high in cholesterol itself, one can see that fish otherwise is quite attractive in its effect on cholesterol levels when compared with meat and fowl.

The Amount of Polyunsaturated Fats in Common Foods

The current recommendations are that **polyunsaturated fats, which currently constitute about 7 percent of calories in the average diet, not be reduced, and can even be increased to 10 percent of calories,** or one-third of the calories obtained from all forms of fat. Foods high in polyunsaturated fats include certain vegetable oils. Vegetable oils are found in cooking and salad oils, fried foods, pastries and other baked goods, margarines, and mayonnaise. Those with a predominance of polyunsaturated fatty acids include safflower oil (75 percent), sunflower oil (66 percent), linseed oil (66 percent), wheat germ oil (62 percent), corn oil (59 percent), soybean oil (58 percent), and cottonseed oil (52 percent).

There are two major types of polyunsaturated fatty acids. One is the omega-6 type. The other is the omega-3 type, found mainly in fish oils (discussed later in the chapter).

The Amount of Monounsaturated Fats in Common Foods

Numerous studies have found that people in certain Mediterranean countries where olive oil is heavily consumed have lower cholesterol levels and less heart disease. The current recommendation is for **monounsaturated fats to constitute 10 to 15 percent of total calories,** or one-third to one-half of calories from all forms of fat. Foods high in monounsaturated fats are certain vegetable oils, here listed with their percentage of monounsaturated fatty acids: olive oil (72 percent), peanut oil (46 percent), and rapeseed (canola) oil (62 percent). (Canola oil is sold under the brand name, Puritan, by Procter & Gamble.) Certain forms of sunflower seed oil and safflower oil (those which are higher in oleic acid than linoleic acid) are more monounsaturated than polyunsaturated. Sesame seed oil has 40 percent monounsaturated fatty acids and 40 percent polyunsaturated fatty acids.

It is wise to reduce the amount of *all* oils in one's food. Nonstick pans are helpful. Spray-on oils or pastry brushes can reduce the amount used to coat pans. Cooking oils should be heated before being added to food. That way, the food will cook faster, and there will be less time for it to absorb the oil. Certain cooking methods use little or no fat and oil: steaming, baking, broiling, grilling, or stir-frying. Foods can be cooked in a microwave oven without having to add fat. When making stews or soups, chill after cooking and skim off the congealed fat from the top after a few hours of cooling in the refrigerator. Try to use nonoil salad dressings (best) or salad dressings made with highly unsaturated or monounsaturated oils (next best). Unsaturated oils should be limited to 6 or 8 tablespoons per day.

Almonds have 75 percent of their fat content in the form of monounsaturated fatty acids. In contrast, English walnuts contain only 27 percent monounsaturated fatty acids, having 62 percent polyunsaturated and 11 percent saturated fatty acids. Nuts in general are relatively high in fat content—most having from 50 to 70 percent fat. Although the fat in nuts is usually unsaturated, their high fat content is reason not to eat them in excess. The fat in avocados is 69 percent monounsaturated. The total fat content of avocados is 16 percent, which is moderate, and less than most meat and dairy products. Broccoli has 13 percent of its calories as fat. Otherwise, most vegetables tend to have between 1 and 7 percent of their calories as fat.

The Omega-3 Fatty Acids in Fish Oils

As mentioned above, one of the two major types of unsaturated acids—the omega-3 fatty acids—are concentrated in fish oils. In addition to lowering cholesterol, these fatty acids tend to reduce the tendency for the blood to clot. This combination of benefits has been thought to reduce heart attacks. Recently, much attention has been directed to the diet of the Greenland Eskimos, who have little in the way of heart disease. Their diet is high in cold-water fish, and contains about seven times the amount of omega-3-fatty acids as the diet of an American eating salmon three times a week. Many researchers believe it is the diet of these Eskimos which is responsible for their low incidence of heart disease. Currently, the omega-3-fatty acids are receiving much attention for their suspected role in reducing cholesterol levels and heart disease.

Why a diet high in fish oils might protect against heart disease remains speculative at this point. Fish, besides being rich in omega-3-fatty acids, has the advantage of being low in saturated fats. Whether it is a diet low in saturated fats or high in omega-3-fatty acids which is responsible for the Greenland Eskimos' low incidence of heart disease is a matter of debate. Some have suggested that their low death rate from heart attacks might be a statistical "artifact" related to the Eskimos' relatively short life span—that is, they do not live long enough to *get* many heart attacks in the first place. Regardless, a number of drug companies have produced and promoted fish-oil supplements which are high in omega-3-fatty acids.

Despite the fact that fish oil supplements are available and are advertised as protective against heart disease, most conservative authorities, including the NHLBI, caution that small amounts of supplements contain too little of the omega-3-fatty acids to do much good, while larger amounts may run the risk of doing harm. Not enough studies have yet been done to determine whether the net effect is beneficial. Fish oil supplements in large amounts have been discovered to cause diabetics to go out of control and to "unmask" borderline diabetes. The fact that Eskimos have twice as many strokes as Danes, with whom they have been compared, raises the fear that high intake of omega-3-fatty acids may excessively lower the tendency for the blood to clot. Recent studies have shown that excessively lowering of the blood's clotting ability can greatly increase the chances of a stroke becoming large (rather than remaining small). One side effect of fish oil capsules is diarrhea, which can occur with only 4 to 6 capsules per day.

Despite the caution about fish oil supplements, most authorities encourage the eating of fish itself at least two to three times a week. A Dutch study has found that this amount of fish can reduce the risk of heart disease significantly. Those interested in increasing their omega-3-fatty acid intake in this way may be curious to see in Exhibit 22–1 how various fish "stack up" in this respect. An easy way to remember which fish are highest in oil content is the color of the meat. The darker the color, the greater the amount of oil, roughly speaking.

Those interested in *canned* fish should be cautioned that canned tuna contains relatively little fish oil compared with fresh tuna. On the other hand, canned sardines and salmon do contain substantially greater amounts of fish oil than canned tuna. Another caution for eaters of canned fish is that processors often add vegetable oil, which can greatly increase the overall fat and caloric content. This can be partly compensated for by draining the oil before eating. Or, you may instead wish to buy fish which is water-packed. Water-packed tuna has the disadvantage of being very bland—the reason why many people add lots of mayonnaise. However, mayonnaise is high in fat, even if that fat is mostly monounsaturated (soybean oil). Lemon or lime juice or low-fat yogurt are better alternative dressings.

Exhibit 22–1   Omega-3 Fatty Acid Content of Fish per 3 Ounce Portion

Extremely High		Very High		High	
Variety	mg	Variety	mg	Variety	mg
Atlantic mackerel	2,500	Atlantic herring	1,600	shrimp	300
		Albacore tuna	1,300	Atlantic cod	300
		Atlantic salmon	1,200	swordfish	200
		bluefish	1,200	haddock	200
				flounder	200

Obesity: A Risk Factor for Disease

Merely being overweight (10 percent above normal) is associated with significantly increased odds of death and disease. In the now-famous Framingham study,* persons who were overweight were found to have *quadruple* the chance of dying over a 30-year period. Besides heart disease and clogged arteries, diseases associated with obesity are diabetes, gout, high blood pressure, gallstones (especially in women), arthritis (because of increased burden on weight-bearing joints), and cancer. Cancer rates among obese people are increased by a third for men and more than a half for women.

But what is "normal"? A quick way to determine one's ideal body weight is to refer to the charts in Exhibits 22–2a and b.

How to Lose Weight

Although the most popular diets are those of the "starvation" type, studies have shown that such diets tend to cause "binging" patterns, which result in weight gain. In addition, repeated crash dieting is associated with *less* weight loss at each subsequent attempt, and progressively *more* weight gain after the diet is abandoned.

The notion that a high-protein diet is the best way to lose weight is a popular fallacy that should be laid to rest. Proof that this notion persists can be ascertained by walking into virtually any restaurant that boasts a "diet plate" on its menu; let's analyze the contents of a typical "diet plate" order:

> One hard boiled egg (sliced into two halves)
> A 6-oz hamburger patty (without bun)
> One scoop cottage cheese
> Several slices or sections of tomatoes
> A leaf of lettuce as decoration, along with
> A few carrot sticks

The carrot sticks, lettuce, and tomatoes are indeed appropriate for a weight-reduction diet. And the egg is not too bad—despite its high cholesterol content—with about 75 calories. However, the cottage cheese, with its high milk-fat content, is rather fattening;

---

*One of the first large-scale studies investigating risk factors for heart disease and death.

Exhibit 22–2a Height and Weight Tables for Men and Women of Average Frame, Ages 25 to 59

Men		Women	
Height	Weight	Height	Weight
5' 2"	131–141	4'10"	109–121
5' 3"	133–143	4'11"	111–123
5' 4"	135–145	5' 0"	113–126
5' 5"	137–148	5' 1"	115–129
5' 6"	139–151	5' 2"	118–132
5' 7"	142–154	5' 3"	121–135
5' 8"	145–157	5' 4"	124–138
5' 9"	148–160	5' 5"	127–141
5'10"	151–163	5' 6"	130–144
5'11"	154–166	5' 7"	133–147
6' 0"	157–170	5' 8"	136–150
6' 1"	160–174	5' 9"	139–153
6' 2"	164–178	5'10"	142–156
6' 3"	167–182	5'11"	145–159
6' 4"	171–187	6' 0"	148–162

Note: Assumes indoor clothing weighing 5 pounds for men and 3 pounds for women, and shoes with 1-inch heels.

Source: Metropolitan Life Insurance Company, copyright 1983. The source of the basic data was *Build Study, 1979*, Society of Actuaries and Association of Life Insurance Medical Directors of America, 1980. Reprinted with permission.

and even worse is the hamburger patty, which—particularly at restaurants, with the grades of meat they tend to choose and the way they usually prepare them (i.e., fried)—is likely to be extremely high in fat. The cottage cheese and hamburger patty are examples of the two most calorie-dense categories of foods: whole-milk dairy products and fried meat products. The only "saving grace" about the "diet plate" is that it might be worse, if it included oily dressings or gravies. Although moderate (but certainly not low) in total calories—having about 750 calories altogether—our sample "diet plate" is not likely to do the dieter much good, because its relatively calorie-dense contents (overall) offer little in the way of long-term satiety. Furthermore, one is likely to break down an hour later and eat something else, such as a rich dessert.

The typical high-protein diet goes astray on two fronts. First,

Exhibit 22–2b   Height and Weight Tables for Men and Women of Average Frame, Ages 60–99

Men		Women	
Height	Weight	Height	Weight
5' 2"	140	4'10"	123
5' 3"	144	4'11"	127
5' 4"	149	5' 0"	130
5' 5"	153	5' 1"	133
5' 6"	158	5' 2"	136
5' 7"	163	5' 3"	140
5' 8"	167	5' 4"	143
5' 9"	172	5' 5"	147
5'10"	176	5' 6"	150
5'11"	181	5' 7"	155
6' 0"	186	5' 8"	158
6' 1"	191	5' 9"	161
6' 2"	196	5'10"	163
6' 3"	200	5'11"	167
6' 4"	207	6' 0"	172

Source: The 1979 Build and Blood Pressure Study covering the years 1954 through 1972 by the Ad Hoc Committee of the New Build and Blood Pressure Study, Association of Life Insurance Medical Directors of America and Society of Actuaries.

most people think of meat products when they think of protein. And, among meat products, they are especially prone to think of hamburger patties. Hamburger patties, in the cheaper grades, contain 20 percent fat—more than in many of the leaner cuts of meat. Indeed, most high-protein foods are admixed with fat; and it is the high fat content that causes obesity. Second, even those high-protein foods that do *not* come admixed with fatty foods, such as soybean products, remain somewhat calorie-dense when compared with fruits, vegetables, and high-fiber foods.

Food Choices for Successful Dieting

The cornerstone of any successful diet requires selecting foods that are *low* in caloric density. This can be portrayed most graphically by realizing that vegetables have only 4 to 12 calories per ounce, whereas chocolate candies, nuts, and cooking oils and fats have from 150 to 250 calories per ounce. Consider, on the one hand, being required to eat a one-pound box of chocolates in a 24-hour period. One could easily finish off the entire box in that time, ending up with 3,200 calories for the day. In contrast, consider being stranded on a desert island for 24 hours with nothing to eat but steamed zucchini. At four calories per ounce, trying to consume the same number of calories as in the one-pound box of chocolates would require consuming 50 pounds of zucchini (about one-third of your body weight)—a physical impossibility.

The above example is, of course, extreme. The point of a low-calorie diet is to limit those foods that are calorie-dense. The most calorie-dense foods are oils and fats, including cocoa fat, which is in chocolates; animal meats, which are high in fat content—especially pork; milk products—especially cream and ice cream, which are extremely high in fat content; and simple sugars, such as table sugar or honey. Fried foods contain large amounts of oil or fat. Most salad dressings are calorie-dense because of the oils they contain—even if those oils are monounsaturated or polyunsaturated. (Nonoil-containing salad dressings are acceptable alternatives.)

The graphs in Exhibit 22–3 enable one to see more readily how certain foods and food groups compare with each other in caloric density.

Diet and Cancer

Estimates are that about 35 percent of all cancers are caused by one's diet (although the range of estimates is from 10 to 70 percent). Certainly, heredity is often a factor. However, if one eliminates heredity, smoking, and occupational hazards, nutrition is left as the single greatest risk for cancer. The following are some of the associations now believed to exist between one's diet and the development of cancer.

Known Associations Between Diet and Cancer

Obesity. Obesity itself—and here we are speaking only of too many *calories*, not of too much *fat* in the diet—has been proved to cause breast cancer in mice. In humans, obesity primarily affects women, such that obese women suffer from an inordinately high

Exhibit 22-3   Calories per Ounce of Some Common Foods

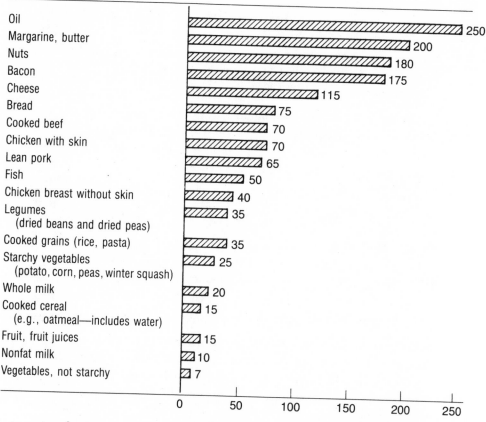

Oil	250
Margarine, butter	200
Nuts	180
Bacon	175
Cheese	115
Bread	75
Cooked beef	70
Chicken with skin	70
Lean pork	65
Fish	50
Chicken breast without skin	40
Legumes (dried beans and dried peas)	35
Cooked grains (rice, pasta)	35
Starchy vegetables (potato, corn, peas, winter squash)	25
Whole milk	20
Cooked cereal (e.g., oatmeal—includes water)	15
Fruit, fruit juices	15
Nonfat milk	10
Vegetables, not starchy	7

rate of certain cancers: breast, cervical, endometrial (the lining of the uterus), ovarian, and gallbladder.

Dietary Fat.   Mice given high amounts of *fat* but not too many *calories* developed more breast cancer. There seems to be a clear association between total fat intake and the development of breast cancer. Much evidence also points to a strong association between total fat intake and the development of colon cancer. In countries where there is a low amount of fat in the diet there tend to be low incidences of both breast and colon cancer. Other cancers associated with a high intake of dietary fat are uterine, ovarian, prostate, pancreas, and gallbladder.

Dietary Fiber.   Dietary fiber seems to have a *protective effect* against the development of colon cancer. For example, rural Scandinavians, even though they have a high-fat diet, have less colon cancer; and this has been attributed to the high amount of fiber in their diet. The "protective effect" of dietary fiber seems to be far less in populations who have a low-fat diet. This suggests that if you must eat a lot of fat, at least try to eat a lot of fiber as well. Still, it is best to eat a diet high in fiber and low in fat. Dietary fiber is also believed to reduce breast cancer. (Fiber is discussed at length later in the chapter.)

Cholesterol Levels.   Suspicion is mounting that a high cholesterol level is associated with colon cancer. The theory is that cholesterol is excreted in the colon via bile acids, which are suspected of playing a role in colon cancer.

Cruciferous Vegetables.   There is fairly strong evidence that certain vegetables have a unique *protective effect* against many of the substances we eat that would otherwise tend to cause cancer. These vegetables increase the normal detoxifying ability of many cells, but especially cells in the liver, where most detoxification takes place. The vegetables are known as "cruciferous" because they have flowers with four leaves in the pattern of a cross. They are primarily Brussels sprouts, cauliflower, broccoli, and cabbage.

Vitamins.   Certain vitamins are suspected of protecting against cancer. The American Cancer Society recommends that people include foods rich in vitamins A and C in their diet. Vitamin A, for example, is suspected of having a protective effect against cancer of the lung, breast, bladder, stomach, esophagus, and larynx. Vitamin A is found in dark green vegetables (spinach, collard, broccoli, green peppers, asparagus), orange-yellow vegetables (pumpkin, squash, carrots, sweet potatoes), orange-yellow fruits (cantaloupe, peaches, apricots), and watermelon. Although vitamin A is also found in milk, cheese, beef, liver, and eggs, such foods tend to be high in fats and/or cholesterol, especially the latter two.

Vitamin C is thought to have a protective effect in humans against cancer of the stomach, esophagus, larynx, and uterine cervix. It may also have a protective effect upon lung cancer as well. Vitamin C is found in citrus fruits, canteloupe, watermelon, papayas, guavas, mangos, strawberries, cabbage, kale, collard leaves, turnip greens, broccoli, Brussels sprouts, cauliflower, potatoes, tomatoes, and peppers.

A word of caution is in order about excessive ingestion of foods high in β-carotene (the precursor of vitamin A), such as carrots.

Sustained ingestion of large quantities of carrots can lead to a condition known as caroteinemia, in which very high levels of β-carotene in the blood cause a reversible orange discoloration of the skin. In addition, one should be warned that a sustained intake of only 25,000 IU (International Units) per day—five times the recommended daily allowance of vitamin A—can cause toxic effects, such as nausea, emotional changes, nosebleeds, headaches, tiredness, leg swelling, and liver enlargement. Very high doses of vitamin C—on the order of 2 to 10 grams per day—can cause kidney stones, diarrhea, an excessively acid blood, and other toxic effects.

Known Cancer-Causing Additives in Food

Certain substances are acknowledged to increase the chances of certain cancers if ingested often enough over long enough periods of time. Compounds called nitrosamines are an example. They tend to be produced from foods which contain nitrites or nitrates, which are commonly used as preservatives, particularly in delicatessen meats. Wood or charcoal smoke contains tars which tend to produce cancer; therefore one should avoid food which has been so exposed. (Thus, the all-American pasttime of "grilling out" is unhealthy, unless the grilling is done with a gas flame.) One should also avoid salt-cured foods, such as ham, bacon, and pork.

Somewhat less of a concern when it comes to causing cancer, and perhaps of greater concern because of allergic kinds of reactions, are various dyes that are added to foods. Examples of items that should be avoided if one wishes to follow a dye-free diet include lipstick, soft drinks, candy, ice cream, toothpaste, and many fruitskins (particularly oranges, which often are artificially dyed).

The Importance of Fiber

Fiber is one of the most important yet most misunderstood aspects of diet. Many people do not realize that there are a number of different *types* of fiber.* Virtually all high-fiber foods are a *mixture* of different types of fiber. Thus, individual high-fiber foods may

---

*Celluloses, hemicelluloses, lignins, pectins, gums, and mucilages.

confer more than one type of health benefit, depending upon which types of fiber they contain.

The Benefits of High-Fiber Foods

The health benefits of a high-fiber diet include lowering choles-terol; preventing cancer, especially colon cancer; losing excess weight; preventing gallstone formation; and reducing problems from diverticular disease, constipation, hemorrhoids, and irritable bowel syndrome. Which benefits one will enjoy is a matter of which fiber-rich foods are eaten.

Lowering Cholesterol. The kinds of fibers that lower blood cholesterol levels are the so-called soluble fibers (so named because they dissolve in water); they include oat bran, pectin, guar, and others. Oat bran can be eaten in the form of oat bran itself (available in health food stores) or in oat products such as oatmeal cereal (made from the germ of the grain) or the newer oat bran cereals now available. Foods high in pectins are carrots, citrus fruits, apples, bananas, and beets. Guar, an emulsifier, is found in processed foods such as commercial ice cream and TV dinners. (One therefore does not pursue sources of guar because the foods it is found in tend to raise cholesterol.) It is important not to confuse oat bran with wheat bran, which contains only 10 percent soluble fiber. In one study, 2 ounces a day of oatmeal (such as 2 cups of hot cereal) or oat bran lowered blood cholesterol 5 percent within six weeks. Other foods high in soluble fiber are prunes, zucchini, corn bran, sweet potatoes, beans, pears, and cauliflower.

Potential drawbacks of pectin and guar (compared with oat bran) are that they slow down the passage of stool, something suspected of increasing one's chances of colon cancer. Oat bran, pectin, and guar have all been found to enhance the development of colon cancer in rats who were fed cancer-producing agents. Overall, though, pectin and guar seem to enhance colon cancer more than oat bran. Because of this effect on the development of colon cancer, it may not be wise to restrict high-fiber foods to those that predominantly contain soluble fiber.

Preventing Cancer. Although other types of high-fiber foods—wheat bran and whole-grain breads and cereals (other than oat products)—have no effect upon cholesterol levels, they are believed to have a strong protective effect upon the development of many cancers, especially colon cancer. These particular foods are high in *insoluble* types of fiber, such as cellulose (found in coarse bran), hemicellulose (found in whole grain breads and cereals), and lignins (found in many fruits and in potatoes).

The association of a lower cancer rate with a high-fiber diet may be indirectly due to the low caloric density of such foods. After being eaten, high-fiber foods absorb water from the body and swell to much more than their original weight. This, in turn, tends to reduce caloric intake, which can reduce obesity (as discussed earlier in this chapter). In addition, high-fiber foods tend to keep blood sugar levels stable (discussed in the next section). The combined effect increases satiety, making it less likely the person will soon be hungry enough to consume other foods, including foods high in fat. Thus, much of the reduction in cancer rate in persons on high-fiber diets may be due to consuming less fat. Eating less fat also reduces the tendency toward obesity.

Controlling Blood Sugar. As mentioned, high-fiber foods tend to be low in caloric density. Besides this, foods rich in soluble fiber (see above) tend to mix with other foods in the stomach and slow their digestion. The result is that blood sugar levels do not rise as rapidly, and there is less tendency for excess insulin to be produced, as often happens after a heavy meal. Without excess insulin, there is less tendency for the "rebound" effect, which commonly occurs some one and a half hours after a large meal. This "rebound effect" is greater the larger the meal, and tends to cause "binging" of a second, though smaller, meal after 1½ to 2 hours. This "second meal" is believed to contribute greatly to weight gain. But when blood sugar levels rise slowly (as with a meal high in soluble fiber), this "rebound effect" does not take place. The person is more likely to remain satiated until the next regular meal, thereby consuming less calories by the end of the day. The result is a trend away from obesity.

Preventing Gallstone Formation. Since most gallstones are formed from cholesterol, a side benefit of a diet higher in soluble fiber (which lowers cholesterol) is less gallstone formation.

Preventing Diverticular Disease. As persons get older, "potholes" tend to form in the large intestine. It is believed that they are caused by the prolonged action, over many decades, of small hard stools. Such stools require more straining, and therefore higher pressure in the colon, to effect passage. This higher pressure is thought to cause weaker portions of the wall of the intestine to "pooch out" into "potholes." A single such "pothole" is called a diverticulum (diverticulae is the plural of diverticulum). The condition of having many of these is called **diverticulosis**. A diet high in insoluble fiber adds bulk to the stool, making it softer and causing it to pass more easily. Such a diet is felt to prevent the formation of diverticulae in the first place. In addition, persons who already have developed the condition of diverticulosis do better on a high-fiber diet, because the stool is softer and easier to pass.

Preventing Constipation and Hemorrhoids. For the same reason that foods high in insoluble fiber cause large bulky stools, constipation is not a problem on a high-fiber diet. Likewise, hemorrhoids—which are largely caused by the straining required to pass small hard stools—tend not to develop.

A Warning About Too Much Fiber

A word of caution is in order for persons who wish to follow a high-fiber diet. Too much fiber too soon can cause abdominal bloating, gas, belching, diarrhea, cramps (sometimes severe), and even bowel blockage. Bowel blockage is most common when supplements, such as bran tablets, are taken in large quantities. It is safest not to use supplements at all, especially bran tablets. But if using bran, a general guide is to begin with only a teaspoon per day and make increases only twice a week. Such increases should be no more than a teaspoon per day. A tablespoon or two per day will eventually suffice in most cases, although some people will benefit from up to two tablespoons three times a day. More than this is excessive, and many people experience side effects from more than a tablespoon or two per day. Unprocessed bran has two grams of fiber in each teaspoonful.

It is best to eat a *variety* of high-fiber foods, containing both soluble and insoluble fibers. And, it is best to use natural foods rather than supplements. People who do choose to use bran are advised to use coarsely ground bran. Finely ground bran tends to defeat the purpose of using bran in the first place and may cause constipation rather than cure it. The current American diet has about 15 to 20 grams of fiber per day. The National Cancer

Institute recommends 20 to 35 grams. More than 55 grams per day is excessive and may cause problems. Despite the fact that wheat bran and all-bran cereal provide some five to six times as much fiber per serving than most other food sources, one should keep in mind that 90 percent of that fiber is of the insoluble type. Thus, by themselves, they do not constitute an ideal high-fiber diet. One should also include sufficient amounts of oat products or various fruits and vegetables which are high in soluble fiber. Some foods that contain more than 50 percent soluble fiber are listed in Exhibit 22–4.

The Importance of Adequate Calcium

Adequate dietary calcium is important to prevent the development of osteoporosis. Osteoporosis is much more of a problem in older women. In our society, females begin to become deficient in calcium intake around age 10 to 14. From then on, their average daily intake declines over the years. At 21, it is less than 700 mg per day. At 75, it is a little over 500 mg per day. In contrast, the daily calcium needs of women increase over the years, being about 1,000 mg per day at 21, 1,200 mg per day during menopause, and 1,500 mg per day after menopause (1,100 mg per day if taking estrogen hormones). Older men, in contrast, require about 800 mg of calcium per day. A rough guide is to consider one portion of any dairy product (such as a glass of milk) as 250 mg, and add 350 mg to the total. If the total is less than 1,000 to 1,500 mg (for women), you may not be getting enough calcium in your diet.

In addition to milk and dairy products (the most common dietary sources of calcium), four vegetables that are especially high in calcium are collards (1 cup cooked, 35 mg), turnip greens (1 cup cooked, 267 mg), kale (1 cup cooked, 206 mg), and mustard greens (1 cup cooked, 193 mg). Seafood high in calcium includes canned salmon and sardines that have the bones still present. A more complete listing of calcium-rich foods can be found in Appendix C.

Certain foods that are high in calcium are of no benefit because they also contain oxalate compounds that block the absorption of calcium. Examples are spinach, swiss chard, beets, and beet greens. Too much fat, fiber, or alcohol tends to reduce the absorption of calcium. Too much phosphorus can also reduce the body's

Exhibit 22–4   Fiber Content in Grams of Natural Foods and Ready-to-
             Eat Cereals

Natural Foods	grams		grams
broccoli ($\frac{1}{2}$ cup)	3.5	Kellogg's Nutri-Grain Wheat	2.0
peach (1 medium)	2.3	Post's Grape-Nuts	2.0
cabbage ($\frac{1}{2}$ cup)	2.1	Wheat Chex	2.0
potato, sweet ($\frac{1}{2}$ medium)	2.1	Kellogg's Nutri-Grain Corn	2.0
apple ($\frac{1}{2}$ large)	2.0	Wheaties	2.0
potato, baked ($\frac{1}{2}$ medium)	1.9	Total	2.0
plums (3 small)	1.8	Cheerio's	2.0
carrots, raw ($\frac{1}{2}$ cup)	1.8	Post's Grape-Nuts Flakes	2.0
orange (1 small)	1.6	Kellogg's Nutri-Grain Wheat & Raisins	1.0
banana ($\frac{1}{2}$ medium)	1.5	Sun Country Granola with Raisins	1.0
apricots (2)	1.4	Life	1.0
grapefruit ($\frac{1}{2}$)	0.8	Raisin Life	1.0
Ready-to-Eat Cereal (per 1-oz Serving)		Almond Delight	1.0
Kellogg's All-Bran with Extra Fiber	13.0	Sun Flakes Crispy Wheat & Rice Flakes	trace
Fiber One	12.0	100% Natural Cereal Raisin & Date	trace
Kellogg's All-Bran	9.0	Crispix	trace
Post's Natural Bran Flakes	5.0	Kellogg's Corn Flakes	trace
Quaker Corn Bran	5.0	100% Natural Cereal	trace
Bran Chex	5.0	Product 19	trace
Nabisco Shredded Wheat 'N Bran	4.0	Kellogg's Special K	trace
Familia Swiss Birchermeusli	4.0	Rice Chex	trace
Kellogg's Bran Flakes	4.0	Rice Krispies	trace
Post's Fruit & Fibre Harvest Medley	4.0	Post's Super Golden Crisp	trace
Post's Fruit & Fibre Mountain Trail	4.0	Corn Chex	trace
Post's Fruit & Fibre Tropical Fruit	4.0	Crispy Wheats 'N Raisins	trace
Kellogg's Fruitful Bran	4.0	Kellogg's Frosted Flakes	trace
Post's Natural Raisin Bran	4.0	Golden Grahams	trace
Cracklin' Oat Bran	4.0		
Familia Genuine Swiss Meusli	3.0		
Nabisco Shredded Wheat	3.0		

ability to absorb calcium; foods high in phosphorus are eggs, red meats, and carbonated drinks.

A high-protein diet—one that contains at least twice the recommended dietary allowance—causes calcium loss. Weight loss also leads to calcium depletion. Too much salt in the diet can cause excessive calcium loss through the urine. Caffeine also promotes calcium loss through the urine; in fact, calcium loss doubles with three cups of coffee per day.

Some persons on low-salt diets may find their diet has little calcium in it because they are avoiding dairy products altogether, on the assumption that all dairy products are high in salt. However, while cheeses tend to be high in salt, milk and yogurt are not.

Certain water pills (diuretics), such as hydrochlorthiazide, tend to *prevent* loss of calcium through the kidneys.

Sugar

For practical purposes there are two basic kinds of sugar: refined sugar, such as table sugar, and unrefined sugar, such as those occurring in fruits. The main problem with refined sugar is that it is absorbed directly into the bloodstream in a rapid manner and has a relatively high caloric density. It therefore does not keep hunger at bay for long, yet it supplies a fair amount of calories. In addition, a moderate amount taken in a short time may lead to overproduction of insulin, which can produce to a "rebound" effect of low blood sugar some one and a half hours later. This low blood sugar tends to cause intense hunger, which can lead to overeating and obesity. Refined sugar also has the drawback of having no nutrient value, thus providing so-called "empty calories."

Refined sugar in moderation, however, does not have any ill effects. The Food and Drug Administration reported in September 1986 that sugar itself did not present a significant public health hazard when consumed at moderate levels.

For people trying to lose weight, the question of artificial sweeteners is of interest. Three types are currently in vogue: cyclamates, saccharine, and aspartame. Cyclamates are now illegal in the United States, and saccharine is illegal in Canada. As one might expect from the fact of their being illegal in one country or another, cyclamates and saccharine are more controversial than aspartame. But even aspartame, commonly known by the brand name Nutra

Sweet, is not 100 percent free of controversy. However, extensive testing has determined that human beings suffer no significant ill effects from ingesting the relatively small amounts of aspartame available in food products.

Salt

A certain amount of hysteria surrounds the use of salt (sodium chloride) in one's diet. There is nothing inherently evil about salt, even in reasonably large amounts. The average American ingests 12 grams of salt per day. On the other hand, certain individuals should limit their salt intake. These are principally persons who suffer from high blood pressure, heart failure, or swollen legs. All those with high blood pressure should limit their sodium intake to about 2 to 3 grams per day. This can be accomplished fairly easily by avoiding foods high in salt and not salting one's food at the table. Patients with congestive heart failure must be stricter, generally limiting sodium to 1 or 2 grams per day. Such severe restriction may require eating specially prepared foods. People who need to avoid salt should try lemon juice or various herbs and spices that also enhance the taste of foods. Persons who wish to use salt substitutes—most of which contain potassium—should check with their doctor first. Some salt substitutes are not completely sodium-free, and actually contain a certain amount of ordinary table salt. Some commonly used foods high in salt are listed in Appendix D.

Caffeine

As with salt, caffeine as a health risk has suffered a degree of unjustified hysteria. Some hasty conclusions were drawn from studies which at first seemed to point to a link between coffee and cancer of the pancreas or benign breast disease. The public may recall the original newspaper headlines better than the subsequent reevaluations which laid these suspicions to rest. However, heavy caffeine intake *has* been found to raise cholesterol levels by as much as 14 percent. And caffeine is known to raise blood pressure and increase stomach acid. Caffeine can produce heart rhythm disturbances in some persons, and has been suspected of contributing to heart attacks. Caffeine—especially three or more cups of coffee per day—can increase calcium loss in the urine.

Caffeine is present in many nonprescription drugs, such as cold remedies, pain pills, stimulants, and appetite suppressants. Although coffee contains the most of any food product (up to 155 mg per cup), other foods also contain caffeine (see Exhibit 22–5).

Iron

Iron is needed by the body chiefly to make red blood cells. Older persons are seldom deficient in iron unless they are ill. Although Geritol has been advertised to older persons as a cure for "tired blood" (and iron deficiency), iron supplements should not be taken by older persons except on the advice of a doctor. Some reasons for a low iron level are discussed in Appendix G. Doctors can detect iron deficiency in various ways. Their methods are discussed in Chapters 3 and 26.

Potassium

Potassium is a salt needed by the body chiefly to help muscle cells contract properly and to transport sugar into the muscles for energy. Potassium deficiency can cause marked weakness and muscle cramping—particularly in often-used muscles such as the calves or the thighs. In persons who are wheelchair-bound, the muscles of the arms or the back of the neck may reflect this deficiency state.

Potassium intake becomes a concern most commonly in persons who are taking "water pills" for conditions such as high blood

Exhibit 22–5   Amount of Caffeine in Drinks and Chocolate

Coffee (1 cup)	up to 155 mg
Tea (1 cup)	up to 50 mg
Cola soft drinks (12 oz)	up to 65 mg
Cocoa (1 cup)	up to 40 mg
Chocolate (1 oz)	6 mg

pressure, heart failure, or leg swelling. Potassium deficiency, and how to correct it, is discussed in some depth in Appendix E.

Vitamins

National standards for vitamins and other nutrients are periodically updated and published by the Food and Nutrition Board of the National Research Council. They are known as the recommended dietary allowances (RDA) and are often referred to on packaging labels. The 1980 revision includes an additional set of recommended allowances for adults over age 50. These RDAs apply only to the average healthy person and may not meet the special needs of everyone. In addition, objections have been raised that they may not be appropriate for the very old—those over age 80.

The best source for vitamins is foods. Persons who eat a well-balanced diet with sufficient calories do not need to take vitamin pills. However, persons who do decide to take vitamins should generally choose a brand that contains close to 100 percent of the RDA of the vitamins it includes. A daily vitamin and mineral supplement may be beneficial for older persons who eat poorly. The RDA levels for the elderly are listed in Exhibit 22–6.

Taking large quantities of certain vitamins, particularly vitamins A, and D, can be dangerous. These vitamins are fat-soluble, and remain stored in body fat and in the liver for longer periods of time. Therefore, they can more easily build up to toxic levels.

There have been many unsubstantiated claims for benefits of vitamin E against heart disease and other ills. Vitamins A and C were discussed earlier in connection with diet and cancer. Those who drink fruit juices as a source of vitamin C should be aware that this vitamin oxidizes rapidly and loses much of its potency (roughly one-quarter to one-half) within a week or two after reconstituted fruit juices are stored in the refrigerator.

Most people are not aware of the importance of the B vitamins (such as folic acid and pyridoxine—B-6) and the fact that they can only be stored to a limited extent. Toxicity is generally not a problem, except perhaps in the case of B-6 when very large quantities are taken in. It is therefore important to include sources of the B vitamins on a daily basis. B vitamins are very sensitive to heat and oxygen. Thus foods that contain them should not be overcooked. Even better is to eat such foods fresh. Good sources

Exhibit 22-6   Recommended Dietary Allowances for People Over Age 50

Protein (g)	56	44
Vitamin A (μg RE)	1000	800
Vitamin D (μg)	5	5
Vitamin E (mg α-TE)	10	8
Vitamin C (mg)	60	60
Thiamin (mg)	1.2	1.0
Riboflavin (mg)	1.4	1.2
Niacin (mg NE)	16	13
Vitamin B_6 (mg)	2.2	2.0
Folacin (μg)	400	400
Vitamin B_{12} (μg)	3.0	3.0
Calcium (mg)	800	800
Phosphorus (mg)	800	800
Magnesium (mg)	350	300
Iron (mg)	10	10
Zinc (mg)	15	15
Iodine (μg)	150	150

Note: Assumes an average weight of 154 pounds for men and 120 pounds for women, and an average height of 70 inches for men and 64 inches for women. The amounts listed are for average people living in the United States under normal conditions. Diets should include a variety of foods to provide these as well as other nutrients for which human requirements are as yet less well defined.

of some of the B vitamins are bananas, spinach, kale, whole grain products, avocados, asparagus, broccoli, Brussels sprouts, potatoes, and sweet potatoes.

Labeling

The current vogue of favoring "natural" or "organic" foods is based on the dangers of food additives. However, purveyors of foods often abuse this term in package advertising, and currently this is not unlawful. One should realize that many foods touted as "natural" or "organic" actually contain the very food additives one might think would be absent. Always look at the list of ingredients to see which additives are present.

Nutrition in the Very Old

Elderly persons—particularly those over 80—are more susceptible to a variety of nutritional deficiencies because of reduced activity and caloric intake. It is more important for them to eat nutritious, well-balanced meals. The most common nutritional deficiencies in the elderly are total calories, calcium, and vitamins A, folic acid, B-6, and C. Vitamin D may be a problem if sun exposure is inadequate (in that vitamin D is synthesized in the skin following sun exposure). Those who tend to eat only small quantities of food may need to have a special diet consisting of high-calorie, nutrient-dense foods.

Foods rich in calcium and vitamins A, B-6, and C were discussed earlier in the chapter. Folic acid (also called "folate") is found in dark green leafy vegetables such as asparagus, broccoli, spinach, kale, mustard greens, beet greens, and Brussels sprouts; in peas, beans, legumes, beets, cabbage, Romaine lettuce, and oranges; in whole grain products; and in the fortified breakfast cereals Product 19 and Total. Special K is fortified only to the 25 percent RDA level and is not as highly recommended.

Some studies have shown magnesium and zinc intake to be inadequate in many of the elderly. A good way to increase these nutrients in the diet is to include more whole fruits instead of fruit juices, and to include whole grain breads and cereals, and dark green leafy vegetables.

Additional alternatives to increase nutrients in the diet are to consume hardy soups made from meat, fish, and fowl, and to add nonfat dry milk powder—particularly for persons who do not drink milk—to various casseroles, soups, and nutritious desserts.

Elderly persons who wish to purchase vitamin supplements might want to compare the ingredients with the recommended dietary allowances for the elderly in Exhibit 22–6.

Those who take folic acid should be aware that folic acid ingestion can mask one important sign of B-12 deficiency—excessive size of the red blood cells (mean corpuscular volume)—which would usually show up on a routine complete blood count. Therefore, it is useful to have at least a complete blood count prior to embarking on vitamin therapy, to try and discern whether you might have a B-12 deficiency. B-12 deficiency in older persons is commonly due to the inability of the stomach to secrete a substance that enables one to properly absorb the B-12 in the diet. Actual dietary deficiency of B-12 itself is extremely rare and for practical purposes occurs only in very strict vegetarians. B-12 deficiency causes damage to the brain and the peripheral nervous system, resulting in problems such as mental confusion and tingling of the hands or feet in severe cases. Past a certain point, much of the damage is irreversible. Caught early, it can be treated easily and before permanent damage occurs by the use of regular vitamin B-12 injections.

One way in which nutrient density can be increased is through the use of nutritional supplements such as Ensure. One problem with nutritional supplements is that they may cause diarrhea in persons who have not been eating for many days. For this reason it may be wise to begin with small quantities. Or, the supplement can be diluted with water to half-strength initially, and increased to full strength as tolerated. If diarrhea persists, switching to a different nutritional supplement, such as Isocal, may solve the problem.

Nutritional supplements are now generally available in supermarkets and pharmacies. If not in stock, they can be special-ordered by the pharmacist. Some of the more popular nutritional supplements are listed in Exhibit 22–7.

Some people who are temporarily ill or who have not eaten for a number of days may develop an intolerance to lactose—the sugar in milk. Such persons may be especially prone to diarrhea. Therefore, they would be advised to avoid not only milk and milk products, but also supplements that contain lactose. The two Meritene products in Exhibit 22–7 contain lactose; the rest do not.

Ensure Plus is especially high in calories, but it is more likely to cause diarrhea. "HN" means high in protein. "HCN" means high

Exhibit 22–7   Nutritional Supplements

Citrotein	Ensure HN
Meritene Liquid	Ensure Plus
Meritene Powder (prepared with whole milk)	Ensure Plus HN
	Isocal
Resource Instant Crystals	Isocal HCN
Enrich	Sustacal
Ensure	Sustacal HC

in both calories and protein. Isocal HCN has twice the calories and protein compared with plain Isocal. Citrotein is more suitable for making punch or jello. Resource Instant Crystals is a powdered form that can be mixed with liquid. It is also now available in ready-to-drink wax cartons. Ensure comes in a variety of flavors.

Most supplements are sold in 6-packs of 8-oz cans, and they are available by the case to save money. For people who have had dental work and are unable to chew temporarily, or who are having some difficulties swallowing, are recuperating from an illness, or are having difficulty shopping, having a ready meal supplement on hand can be important in maintaining one's nutrition. Each can has a complete complement of all the essential nutrients. For an average person, about six 8-oz cans per day will provide all the calories and nutrients needed. About three cans per day should suffice for persons who eat 50 percent of their usual diet.

Some elderly persons eat so little that tube feedings are necessary. Tube feedings are usually instituted in a hospital setting. An x-ray is taken after placement of the tube to be sure that it has passed down to the stomach, and not into the lungs. Nutritional supplements such as Ensure are able to satisfy all nutritional requirements except for some additional water in certain cases. (The ethical aspects of tube feedings are discussed in Chapter 29.)

The Interaction of Drugs and Food

Most people are aware that many drugs interact with each other, and with alcohol, and they are especially cautious (as they should be) about drinking alcohol without a doctor's advice if they are taking medication. However, drugs also interact with foods, and in numerous ways. One of the most common examples is the effect of the thiazide diuretics (such as hydrochlorthiazide—also sold under the brand name of Hydrodiuril), which cause potassium loss, although they also tend to prevent loss of calcium. Another common food-drug interaction is the effect of food—especially milk products—on the absorption of the antibiotic tetracycline. This antibiotic is absorbed well only if taken at least an hour before or an hour and a half after meals. In general, though, it is best to take drugs with meals or immediately after, or with a small amount of food, such as a piece of toast or a glass of milk, to avoid the tendency of many drugs to upset the stomach. Even when drugs do not cause frank nausea or stomach upset, they may often cause loss of appetite—particularly when there are many drugs which must be taken at the same time. The American Dietetic Association has an excellent handbook on the interaction of drugs and foods.*

*Daphne A. Roe, *Interaction of Selected Drugs and Nutrients* (The American Dietetic Assn., 1982).

Chapter 23

SMOKING

Working at the hotel was what really made me change my attitude about smoking. I saw how the ones who smoked were like living death—they could not even walk around the block. Everyone should work at a senior citizens' hotel when they are young so they can see what happens when you get old if you do not take care of yourself. One week there would change your life; you would have to be crazy for it not to.

This comment, from a desk clerk at a senior citizens' residence hotel, is a convincing statement in the case against cigarette smoking. So is the surgeon general's summary of the risk of smoking: "Cigarette smoking is the chief, single avoidable cause of death in our society and is the most important public health issue of our time." And the House of Delegates of the 1986 American Academy of Family Practice has called on family doctors to make the cessation of smoking the number one priority in their practices.

Deaths from the use of tobacco in this country are now pegged at about 350,000 per year—more than the total number of Americans killed in World War I, the Korean War, and the Vietnam War combined. The annual cost is $65 billion dollars—$22 billion for direct medical costs, and $43 billion in lost earnings and productivity.

Smoking: Hazardous to Your Health

Most people think of smoking as something not to do only because it causes lung cancer. However, many people do not realize that

212

smoking has a devastating effect on one's health for a variety of other reasons, as well.

Smoking and Cancer

In addition to being linked to lung cancer, smoking is associated with 30 percent of *all* cancers. Here are some facts on smoking's role in cancer:

Lung Cancer. Smoking causes 85 percent of all deaths from lung cancer. Persons who smoke are 14 times more likely than nonsmokers to die of lung cancer. The chances of getting lung cancer increase with the number of cigarettes smoked, how much one inhales, how many years one smokes, and the tar and nicotine content of the cigarettes smoked. Having started smoking at an early age is also an important factor; men who began smoking before age 15 have a death rate from lung cancer four times more than men who did not begin smoking until after age 25. Those who smoke pipes and cigars have a considerably lower rate of lung cancer than those who smoke cigarettes, but their rate is still greater than in nonsmokers.

Cancer of the Larynx. Men are 16 times, and women 9 times, more likely to develop cancer of the larynx if they smoke. The risk is no less among those who smoke pipes or cigars instead of cigarettes. Those who also drink have an even higher risk, because the chemicals in cigarette smoke that cause cancer dissolve in alcohol, and the alcohol enables the chemicals to penetrate the tissues more readily.

Mouth Cancer. Cancers of the lip, tongue, floor of the mouth, and other areas of the mouth are 3 to 10 times more common in cigarette smokers compared with nonsmokers. For those who also drink heavily, the risk increases from 6 to 15 times. Pipe and cigar smoking, as well as tobacco chewing, also causes cancer at various locations in the mouth.

Cancer of the Esophagus. Smokers have an increased risk of death of 2 to 9 times compared with nonsmokers, depending on the amount of alcohol they imbibe.

Cancer of the Pancreas. Death from this cancer is double in smokers in general, and is five times as great in males who smoke more than two packs per day. Of course, persons who smoke often tend to drink as well, so this association may be at least partially due to the drinking of alcohol.

Cancer of the Kidneys and Bladder. The risk of cancer of the kidneys is increased from 1-½ to 2-½ times for smokers. The increased risk of bladder cancer is more than seven times as great in smokers, and ten times as great in heavy smokers. In addition, 40 percent of all bladder cancers in males, and 31 percent of all bladder cancers in females, are linked to cigarette smoking.

Cancer of the Cervix. Women who smoke have an increased incidence of cancer of the cervix.

Ill Effects Other Than Cancer

In addition to causing cancer, smoking shortens life in other ways. Overall, smokers live 8.3 years less than nonsmokers. Chronic lung disease is a major problem with smokers. Other health problems are linked to smoking as well.

Chronic Lung Disease. Technically termed **chronic obstructive pulmonary disease**, chronic lung disease is the fourth leading cause of death in persons 65 and over.

Chronic lung disease consists of two kinds of problems: bronchitis and emphysema. **Bronchitis** is the inflammation of the mid-sized breathing passageways in the lungs. **Emphysema** is the destruction of the architecture and elastic abilities of the smallest air passages and lung sacs, resulting in reduced ability to move air. Emphysematous changes are essentiallly irreversible, while changes from bronchitis are reversible to a certain extent. Both conditions predispose to pneumonia.

Cigarette smoking is the leading cause of chronic bronchitis and emphysema. Smokers have an increased death rate from chronic lung disease of 4 to 25 times that of nonsmokers. Ninety percent of chronic bronchitis and emphysema cases are caused by cigarette smoking.

Persons in the final stages of chronic lung disease get so short of breath that they have difficulty accomplishing ordinary tasks involved in daily living, such as dressing, bathing, cooking their meals, and particularly going shopping or climbing stairs. Some of these people can live an extra year or two by breathing in oxygen for at least 12 to 18 hours per day. They often need special assistance from a team of health professionals, including a respiratory therapist, physical therapist, dietician, and visiting nurse, to enable them to continue independent living as long as possible before ending up in a nursing home. Most would benefit from annual flu shots and from the pneumonia vaccine (discussed in Chapter 27).

An important fact about chronic lung disease is that it often occurs silently—usually developing over a period of 10 or more years—without the affected persons becoming aware of it until they develop serious impairment, such as a chronic cough, wheezing, or shortness of breath. Most persons are diagnosed between the ages of 55 and 65. By then, however, it is really too late to reverse the damage that has occurred. For this reason, it is important that all cigarette smokers—including those who may have quit—past the age of 35 have certain lung function tests, called "spirometry," and continue to have such tests at least every five years. This lung test can be done in the doctor's office, although not all doctors have the equipment and may refer their patients to the respiratory therapy department of a hospital. Spirometry consists of taking in a deep breath and breathing into a tube as hard and completely as possible. Measurements on a machine connected to the tube tell the doctor whether a significant amount of chronic lung disease has already developed, and if so, how bad it has become. Of course, the main purpose in identifying whether a person has developed some degree of chronic lung disease is to warn them that they are at particularly high risk for early death and a disabling, downhill course if they continue to smoke, or resume smoking.

Heart Disease. Along with high blood cholesterol and high blood pressure, smoking is one of the three major risk factors for heart attacks and sudden death from heart disease. With all three risk factors present, the death rate from heart disease is 300 percent greater. With cigarette smoking alone, the death rate is 60 percent greater.

Clogged Arteries. Smoking is a major cause of clogged arteries, whether to the heart or elsewhere in the body.

Strokes. According to the American Cancer Society, smokers are three times more likely to die of a stroke.

High Blood Pressure. Although smoking has not yet been accepted as a definite risk factor for high blood pressure, it remains suspect. In one study in England, two cigarettes and 200 mg of caffeine produced an average systolic blood pressure rise of 18 and a diastolic rise of 8 within an hour.

Osteoporosis. Smoking tends to cause earlier menopause in women. By this mechanism it is felt to be responsible for an increase in brittle bones in later life in women who smoke.

Peptic Ulcer Disease. Various studies have found that smokers run a one and a half to two times greater risk of getting stomach and duodenal ulcers.

Deaths from Fires. Cigarettes are the leading cause of fatal fires. About one out of five fires in the United States is caused by cigarette smoking.

The Benefits of Quitting

Assuming that you are sufficiently convinced by all of the above facts to stop smoking, you may be encouraged to know that some of the bad effects of cigarette smoking are reversible, in time. Statistics show that the risk of death from heart disease reverts back to that of nonsmokers after 10 years. In the case of bladder cancer, the risk reverts back after only 7 years. For cancer of the larynx, it takes 10 years. For lung and mouth cancer, it takes from 10 to 15 years. Figures are not available for the remaining cancers and conditions that are made worse by smoking, but in all cases there is improved risk after smoking is stopped.

How to Quit: It's Not Easy

The latest figures* show that 26 percent of adults continue to smoke—a considerable drop from previous years. These figures may encourage the remaining smokers to stop when they realize they are no longer in the majority and it is no longer socially acceptable to smoke.

---

*"Progress in Chronic Disease Prevention: Cigarette Smoking in the United States, 1986," *Journal of the American Medical Association* 258, no. 14 (Oct. 9, 1987), 1877–81.

However, as most smokers know, it is not easy to stop. Of those who try, about 25 to 30 percent resume smoking within a year. The reason is due in large part to the nicotine in cigarettes, which has been compared to cocaine in the strength of its addicting qualities. It is believed that those who have already quit smoking were relatively light smokers, and that the remaining smokers are largely heavy smokers who will find it more difficult to quit.

Many methods are currently available to help smokers quit. Some rely on psychological techniques; others use a combination of such techniques with chemical aides such as nicotine gum or drugs designed to ease the symptoms of withdrawal.

Psychological Techniques

It has been found that much more success is achieved by those who quit "cold turkey," compared with those who gradually try to cut down a little at a time. Likewise, more success is achieved by those who undergo a formal program with professional assistance, compared with those who try to stop "on their own." Many of these programs have the participants sign a "contract" to stop smoking by a specified date and award a printed certificate upon successful completion of the program. The American Academy of Family Practice and the American Society of Internal Medicine have kits that doctors can use to assist their patients to quit smoking. In addition, self-help printed and audiovisual materials are available to smokers from the American Lung Association, the American Heart Association, and the federal government (see Chapter 31).

Chemical Aids

Nicotine gum is available by prescription under the name Nicorette. It is one of the more successful aids to smoking cessation. It is most successful when used in a structured program under a doctor's supervision (rather than just "handed out"). The gum is chewed repeatedly during the day to relieve the withdrawal symptoms of nicotine addiction. These symptoms may include irritability, anxiety, headache, restlessness, poor concentration, and stomach or intestinal distress.

Other prescription drugs that have been used to relieve the physical symptoms of nicotine withdrawal are various tranquilizers, antidepressant drugs, and certain high blood pressure medications which have also been used with some success in treating cocaine addicts. One of the most successful of the latter is clonidine (Catapres). It is typically prescribed in doses of 0.1 mg at bedtime, and 0.05 mg at other times of the day, as needed, up to a daily total of 0.2 mg.

Chapter 24

DRINKING

In recent years, several studies have suggested that the moderate use of alcohol may have beneficial effects on the heart—perhaps tending to prevent heart disease. It is understandable that such studies in support of moderate drinking are quoted by manufacturers of alcoholic beverages and by those who drink. However, the reader should be cautioned that all the studies done thus far have been quite limited and that no authoritative groups have rallied to the use of alcohol as a way of preventing heart disease. The information we have so far is inconclusive.

This is not to say that alcohol, in moderation, is either good or bad. At this time, we just do not know. What is clear is that the *abuse* of alcohol in the United States is known to cause about 100,000 deaths per year and to result in economic costs of $120 to $150 billion for medical treatment, motor vehicle accidents, lost jobs, and so forth.

The Potential Dangers of Daily Alcohol Use

When doctors caution against the use of alcohol for possible benefits against heart disease, they often refer to its potential "dangers." Few people need to be convinced of the dangers of alcoholism—that is, clearly excessive use. What most people are perhaps not aware of are the *insidious* dangers of daily alcohol use at a level that falls short of frank alcoholism. The problem is that many changes go unnoticed until they reach an advanced state, when it is too late to correct much of the damage that has been done.

Effects of Alcohol on the Body

The ravages of alcohol affect virtually every part of the body. Many people think of alcohol as affecting only the liver—the organ that metabolizes alcohol and suffers much of its toxic effects. However, alcohol also has wide-ranging effects on the heart, the brain, the nerves in the arms and legs, the muscles, the pancreas, the stomach, the bones, and the lungs—just to mention a few.

The Heart.   One of the most important effects of alcohol on the heart stems from an increase in blood pressure. Drinking may be the single most correctable cause of high blood pressure. Even light to moderate drinking—but certainly more than three drinks per day—can increase blood pressure, an effect which typically lasts for several days. The effect of alcohol on blood pressure subsides after a week. Drinking increases the heart rate. With prolonged excessive drinking, the heart muscle weakens, and there is a tendency for erratic beating. Such problems can be life-threatening.

The Brain.   The milder effects of alcohol on the brain include short-term memory loss (although there is a lesser degree of long-term memory loss, as well). Sufficient heavy drinking over many years produces dementia. The part of the brain which controls balance is affected. This, in turn, leads to repeated falls, which often result in broken bones. There is an increase in fatal strokes in heavy drinkers. Many older persons have problems falling asleep and use a "nightcap" to help them fall asleep faster. The problem here is that, while alcohol may help them *fall* asleep, the *quality* of the subsequent sleep is poor. This results in irritability and lethargy the following day.

The Nerves to the Arms and Legs.   The legs are affected much more than the arms. Part of the nerves are destroyed, leading to numbness below a certain point, as if the person were wearing stockings which cause a loss of sensation beneath them.

The Muscles.   Prolonged excessive drinking leads to weakness from shriveling up of the skeletal muscles. Typically, this happens with more than 3-½ oz of alcohol per day consumed for more than three years.

The Pancreas. Although it remains a mystery just how, why, and when problems in the pancreas arise, persons with a history of heavy drinking tend to develop attacks of inflammation of the pancreas (called **pancreatitis**). These attacks can occur not just during bouts of heavy drinking, but even years after drinking has stopped. The person typically develops severe abdominal pain, nausea, and vomiting. Such attacks often require hospitalization in order to provide supportive care, such as suctioning the stomach, intravenous fluids, and pain shots, so the pancreas can rest. Bouts of pancreatitis typically last about a week, and may recur months or years later. In some persons, a low-grade inflammation of the pancreas persists, causing continual pain and digestive difficulties for extended periods of time.

The Stomach. Excessive drinking can cause inflammation of the stomach, which can lead to serious blood loss from the irritated tissues. Heavy drinking often causes ulcers of the stomach or duodenum or varicose veins in the esophagus. Such varicose veins are common in heavy drinkers after several decades of abuse. These may ulcerate and produce heavy, life-threatening episodes of bleeding.

The Bones. Persons who drink excessively tend to develop brittle bones in later life, for a variety of reasons. Strong bones depend on adequate dietary intake of calcium, vitamin D, and phosphates. Heavy drinkers tend to be deficient in their intake of these nutrients in their diets, and their metabolism is affected so that what little they do take in is not properly used. It is suspected that proper absorption does not take place in the stomach and the intestines. The heavy use of antacids common among drinkers tends to interfere with phosphorus absorption. Phosphates are also lost through vomiting and diarrhea—problems that tend to plague heavy drinkers. There is impairment in heavy drinkers of the metabolism of vitamin D to the active form, which takes place in the kidneys. In men, the toxic effects of alcohol on the testicles alters the production of certain hormones which normally stimulate bone formation. A rather strange problem common to heavy drinkers is destruction of part of the thigh bone where it inserts into the hip joint. This problem is felt to be a combination of the effects of alcohol upon the circulation, the bones, and various hormones.

The Lungs.   Heavy drinking impairs the immune system. This, in turn, is believed to be responsible for the marked increase in the incidence of pneumonia and tuberculosis that plagues alcoholics.

Other Organs.   Prolonged drinking can lead to loss of body hair (in the armpits, for example), enlargement of the breasts, and shrinking of the testicles in men. Commonly, there is a tendency to lose potassium. Low potassium can cause muscle weakness and disturbances of the heart rhythm. It can cause additional problems in the cases of persons who might develop high blood pressure or heart failure—conditions for which doctors often use "water pills" as a treatment. With a tendency to potassium loss already present, the use of water pills—which can cause further potassium loss— becomes more of a problem. Drinking causes an increase in the level of fats in the blood. This is because alcohol consists of "empty calories," which turn directly to fat. The effect lasts for up to 36 hours after drinking is stopped. The incidence of cancers in the head and neck are more common in heavy drinkers. A certain type of anemia—caused by a vitamin deficiency (folic acid)—is common in heavy drinkers. Gout attacks are more common in heavy drinkers because alcohol reduces the ability of the kidneys to clear uric acid from the bloodstream.

Drugs That Interact with Alcohol

In addition to all of the above problems that alcohol can cause, one should include the interaction of drugs with alcohol. This problem is of particular importance to senior citizens, since many of them require one or more drugs for various medical conditions.

One of the most dangerous reactions can occur between alcohol and various pills for diabetes, such as chlorpropamide (Diabinese). These can cause nausea and vomiting and other symptoms, even with a single drink. On rare occasions, such reactions are life-threatening. Various drugs for diabetes can also result in low blood sugar, in conjunction with alcohol use.

The sleeping pill chloral hydrate, when used with alcohol, can cause marked dilatation of the blood vessels, which reduces blood pressure. This condition can be especially dangerous when one first stands up, and may result in fainting. Most high blood pressure pills, certain types of pills for depression (the so-called tricyclic antidepressants), and nitroglycerine produce an even greater tendency for the blood pressure to fall, when combined with alcohol. This can cause fainting or falling if the blood pressure gets too low.

Aspirin, which is itself irritating to the stomach, is even more irritating when combined with alcohol, and it may cause internal bleeding. Increased drowsiness or even severe depression of the central nervous system (i.e., coma or semi-coma) can occur when alcohol is combined with certain cold pills, narcotic pain pills, nerve pills, sleeping pills, or pills for depression. Particularly in the case of barbiturates, many inadvertent deaths have occurred in persons who were not aware of this combined effect, and took a large number of them while heavily intoxicated.

How Much Drinking Is Too Much?

With more awareness of the dangers of excessive drinking, readers may begin to wonder about themselves, a friend, or a relative. Is her drinking excessive? Is my drinking excessive? Physicians—especially those with experience in treating alcoholics—can help answer this question. Certainly, drinking is excessive if it disrupts one's job or personal life. On the other hand, what about those who do not suffer any disruption in their lives, yet wonder if their daily consumption of alcohol is slowly eroding away their brain, pancreas, bones, liver, immune system, blood cells, and other organs? For those who would like objective information which bears on this question, there are certain telltale blood tests. Particularly important is the size of the red blood cells (measured during a "complete blood count"); they tend to increase in size in persons who drink too much. Such tests are relatively inexpensive. Other telltale tests are certain enzymes produced in excessive amounts by the liver. These tests can provide useful clues when one is trying to decide whether alcohol consumption is excessive. Besides blood tests, four questions are widely used by doctors who treat alcoholics, in order to determine if the person may suffer from alcoholism. These questions are referred to as the "CAGE Questionnaire":

C—Have you ever felt you should *Cut* down on your drinking?

A—Do you get *Annoyed* when people criticize you for drinking?

G—Have you ever felt *Guilty* about your drinking?

E—Have you ever had an *"Eye-opener"* the first thing in the morning to get rid of a hangover or steady your nerves?

Answering "yes" to two or more of the above questions is believed to indicate a strong possibility of a serious problem with alcohol.

How Elderly Alcoholics Are Different

Many alcoholics who begin drinking heavily in their 20s and 30s do not survive past the age of 60. Young alcoholics have a very high rate of death from cirrhosis of the liver, cancer, accidents, and suicide. For this reason, there are not nearly as many elderly alcoholics. Beyond this, however, doctors have noted a distinct difference between persons who *begin* to drink heavily in their later years—between 40 and 60—and those who began to drink heavily before age 40. The former—that is, the "late-onset" alcoholics—tend to drink in response to specific stresses in life, such as death of a spouse or loneliness, rather than out of sheer compulsiveness. Such "late-onset" alcoholics have been found to be more "treatable" and to have a higher "cure" rate once they receive therapy for their drinking problem. It should be mentioned that the key to a successful "cure" from alcoholism is total abstinence, rather than trying to cut down slowly.

It is not clear precisely how many senior citizens have drinking problems, but one study found alcoholism present in 2.2 percent of persons 65 to 74, and in 1.2 percent of persons 75 and older. Alcoholics who are 60 and older are more likely than younger alcoholics to be divorced, separated, or widowed, and much more likely to be living alone. The single group of elderly most prone to alcoholism are widowers; one study found 10.5 percent of such men to have a serious alcohol problem. Despite these relatively small figures, one study found 82 percent of arrests in elderly persons to be for public drunkenness. In addition, alcoholism among the elderly has been found to comprise 20 percent of nursing home residents and up to 50 percent of persons admitted to psychiatric hospitals.

Because older alcoholics are less likely to have florid withdrawal symptoms or go into "D.T's," or even to show frank signs of intoxication, their drinking problems are often missed by their doctors. This problem is not made easier by the fact that alcoholics tend to minimize greatly the amount they drink. The mental confusion sometimes present in elderly alcoholics may be mistaken by doctors as a sign of dementia, and signs of psychosis caused by alcohol are sometimes diagnosed as mental problems. Therefore, it is useful if relatives or friends can provide an older person's doctor with information about the true amount of alcohol consumed.

Various support organizations, such as Alcoholics Anonymous, can provide assistance and information for persons who have a problem with alcohol. These are listed in Chapter 30.

Chapter 25

EXERCISE

One recurring theme in this book is that various habits affect one's health in a wide variety of ways. For example, a proper diet can reduce one's chances of heart attacks, brittle bones, and many cancers. In the case of exercise, an even wider array of health benefits accrue. Indeed, there has been a tendency to praise exercise as a panacea to improve the memory, relieve constipation, end insomnia, and provide a host of other wide-ranging benefits. As for the risks, there are two schools of thought. One tends to minimize the dangers, claiming that sudden deaths in older persons who were exercising have merely been coincidences—that is, they would have occurred at that moment, no matter what the person was doing. The other school insists on the importance of everyone over 35 having a complete health checkup by a doctor, with an EKG and exercise testing, before even thinking about changing from a sedentary life-style to one that includes a regime of active exercise. Recently, research in these areas was reviewed to determine just which claims are credible and which are not.*

The Benefits and Risks of Exercise

Benefits of Exercise

In certain areas, research has clearly established the benefits of exercise, among them the following:

*Phelps, J.R. "Physical Activity and Health Maintenance—Exactly What Is Known?" *Western Journal of Medicine* (1987) Feb: 146:200–206.

Reduced Risk of High Blood Pressure. Persons who are sedentary run a 35 to 52 percent greater chance of developing high blood pressure, compared with those who keep active. Exercise not associated with work seems to be more beneficial than activity performed on the job.

Reduced Risk of Obesity. In general, exercise tends to reduce the likelihood of becoming obese, as well as to reduce weight in persons who are obese to begin with. Doctors speak of something called "lean body mass," meaning a person's theoretical weight without any fat whatsoever. A certain amount of fat is necessary and healthy. However, beyond this, the rest is excessive. Exercise tends to eliminate a person's "excess fat" and to reduce the weight of obese persons closer toward their "lean body mass."

Exercise is often recommended by doctors in conjunction with a change in diet in treating obesity. When persons have become used to eating a certain diet, it is difficult to make radical changes in their diet in order to achieve weight loss. However, adding an exercise program will "burn up" a certain amount of calories and allow obese patients more latitude in their diet. To take an extreme example: An obese person could continue to eat the same number of calories per day as previously and lose weight merely by exercising much more. However, the most successful programs combine a change to a *moderate* and sensible diet with a program of *moderate* exercise (assuming the person previously had been sedentary).

Reduced Incidence of Heart Disease and Clogged Arteries. The benefits of exercise are clear, especially for persons who also have other risk factors, such as high blood pressure, smoking, obesity, or a family history of heart and clogged artery problems.

Increased Self-Esteem. Here, the benefits seem to accrue more from aerobic activities (described later in the chapter).

Reduced Risk of Osteoporosis. Numerous studies have shown that exercise increases bone density, thereby tending to prevent the osteoporosis that often comes with advancing age (see Chapter 9).

Reduced Risk of Colon Cancer. It has been clearly shown that men who have sedentary occupations tend to get colon cancer more than men who are physically active in their jobs.

Unproven Benefits of Exercise

In certain areas, research has so far *failed* to show any definite benefits from exercise. In other areas there is at least *some* evidence that exercise is beneficial, but the evidence is either weak or there are conflicting reports.

Smoking Cessation. It has not yet been demonstrated that exercising helps a person to quit smoking, or that persons who exercise are less likely to take up the habit. Nevertheless, exercise is often recommended as an aid to smoking cessation.

Improved Mental Functioning. Exercise has not yet been shown to improve memory or thinking ability.

Improved Sleep. Although one study showed that physically active persons thought they slept better, no objective studies (such as those using brain wave measurements) have yet demonstrated such a benefit.

Prevention of Diabetes. Although exercise is clearly known to have a beneficial effect on diabetics who take insulin, no studies have yet shown that regular exercise prevents persons from getting diabetes in the first place. Still, strong suspicion remains that there may be such a benefit.

Less Constipation. Despite the common belief, even among doctors, that exercise promotes regularity, no good studies have yet been done to provide hard evidence that this is so. There has been very little research done in this area.

Improved Blood Tests Relating to Cholesterol. Numerous studies have been done which, overall, tend to suggest that exercise improves certain blood tests relating to cholesterol. These test results, in turn, have been associated with less heart disease and clogged arteries.

Reduced Risk of Anxiety and Depression. Not many studies have been done in this area, and there are some conflicting reports. However, there does seem to be some evidence that exercise reduces anxiety and tends to prevent depression.

Risks of Exercise

Research has clearly established two areas of concern for senior citizens who exercise: injuries and sudden death.

Injuries. There is no question that sports injuries do occur. They are clearly related to the intensity of the exercise, the frequency of exercising, and the length of the workouts. In one study of competitive long-distance runners, a third suffered some kind of injury within a year.

Sudden Death. The myth that athletes develop immunity to heart disease has now been disproved. A study of vigorous men showed that they had a seven-fold higher risk for sudden death while pursuing intense exercise than while they were not exercising. However, their overall risk of sudden death was still found to be *only a third* of the risk for men who were always sedentary. So, overall, it seems to be quite worthwhile to exercise.

The Importance of Exercise Screening

Because the risk of sudden death increases while exercising, it is wise, even for apparently healthy persons older than 35, to undergo a medical evaluation before pursuing a program that will require a major increase in physical activity. With gradual increases in activity, there is only minimal risk. However, certain persons should seek medical advice, even before pursuing *gradual* increases in activity. These include persons with any of the following problems:

- important general medical conditions, such as diabetes
- uncontrolled high blood pressure
- unknown blood pressure
- problems with the joints, such as arthritis
- a family history of heart problems at an early age
- pains around the heart during or immediately after exercise— including pains in the neck, left shoulder, or arm
- a history of heart trouble
- spells of severe dizziness or frequently feeling faint

A medical evaluation can often discover dangers to vigorous activity; also, a person can be advised about an appropriate level of activity to pursue. A subsequent test can evaluate a person's *response* to an exercise program.

A medical evaluation involves, besides a physical examination, a review of the person's individual and family history of heart disease and other risk factors such as high blood pressure, obesity, smoking, and high cholesterol level. A resting EKG is performed. In addition, certain exercise tests are performed in an attempt to discover any latent signs or symptoms of heart disease. Typical tests involve exercising on a treadmill or a stationary bicycle. An older method of exercise testing that is still widely used is repeatedly stepping up and down on a box consisting of two steps; EKG monitoring is continuously performed before, during, and afterward.

Just as in vigorous exercise, there is an increased risk of sudden death merely from undergoing exercise testing. Studies have shown this risk to be less than 1 per 10,000. Less-than-fatal heart problems which require hospitalization occur about 2.4 times per 10,000 tests. The exercise test is halted if the person develops symptoms, such as chest pain, while undergoing the test, or if there are abnormal "squiggles" on the EKG.

Exercise Programs

To be effective, exercise must be done at least three times a week, last at least 15 to 30 minutes, and be of sufficient intensity to increase the pulse and rate of breathing. Workouts should include at least a 5-minute period of "warm-up" exercises beforehand and a 5-minute period of "cooling-down" afterward. The warm-up period should include stretching exercises for the muscles that will be used and a gradual increase in activity. The "cooling-down" period is one of gradual reduction in activity. For example, after a period of running, the person should change to a gradually slowing walk the last 5 minutes. The warm-up exercises are important to reduce the chances of injuries and overexertion. The "cool-down" exercises are important to prevent pooling of blood in the legs, which can lead to passing out or other heart problems if one stops vigorous exercise suddenly.

Exercise regimens should increase gradually. The guidelines of the American Heart Association (AHA) are to try to exercise to the point where the heart beats between 60 and 75 percent of its maximum rate. (The first few months you should restrict yourself to the 60 percent level; after six months you are allowed to go as high as 85 percent.) The maximum heart rate (the 100 percent level) averages 220 minus your age. Exhibit 25–1 contains some

Exhibit 25–1   Maximum Heart Rate and Target Zone for Various Ages

Age	Maximum Heart Rate	Target Zone
45	175	105–131
50	170	102–127
55	165	99–123
60	160	96–120
65	155	93–116
70	150	90–113

Source: American Heart Association.

values for the maximum heart rate and the AHA's "Target Zone" for various ages.

Persons who take medications regularly should be aware that certain preparations for high blood pressure can affect the maximum heart rate. The following medicines tend to *slow* the peak heart rate: Catapres (clonidine), Aldomet (methyldopa), Minipress, and verapamil (Calan and others). The following medicines tend to *increase* the peak heart rate: hydralazine, nifedipine, and nitrates (such as Isordil).

Types of Exercise

Several categories of exercise can be performed. Exercises that require significant oxygen use (and which tend to cause an increase in the respiratory rate) are known as **aerobic exercises.** Running, swimming, and calisthenics are examples. They tend to be exercises which require continuous effort without rest periods. Aerobic exercises are also known as "slow, long-distance" activities.

Exercises that require little oxygen use and therefore do not tend to increase the respiratory rate are known as an **anaerobic exercises.** An example is weight-lifting. Exercises that involve no movement of body parts but merely pressing against a fixed object are called **isometric exercises.** (They are a form of anaerobic exercise.) Older persons are cautioned against engaging in isometric exercises, which have an increased danger of bad effects, such as passing out or raising the blood pressure. They are not recommended by the President's Council on Physical Fitness and Sports. Aerobic exercises confer more cardiovascular benefits, and therefore are of greater benefit than anaerobic exercises to older persons.

General Cautions

Some general rules for exercising are never to exercise under extremes of temperature or in icy conditions, avoid sudden twisting motions, and avoid exercise that might tax your powers of vision or balance. You should avoid competitive sports when starting out if you are a type of person who might not be able to control the natural urge to overtax yourself. You should avoid such extremes of exertion that make you more than pleasantly tired the day after. You should not exercise when ill, such as with a viral infection or a cold. You should avoid very warm temperatures immediately after a workout, such as a very hot shower.

Avoiding the Pitfalls of Doom and Gloom

A common pitfall is to avoid exercise altogether, for fear of getting a heart attack, and for fear that anything less than a vigorous exercise program will not be beneficial. In fact, even light exercise, such as gardening, confers great benefit. Light exercise, even *one half hour a day* more than sedentary persons gets, has been found to reduce heart trouble by a third and death from heart attacks by 70 percent! This type of exercise can be accomplished by just going for a half-hour walk once a day, or a 15-minute walk twice a day. For the vast majority of people, it is not necessary to see a cardiologist just to be able to safely go for a walk.

Chapter 26

THE COMPLETE PHYSICAL

Older persons often reply to their doctor's suggestion to have a "complete physical" with the reply that they "feel fine—so what's the point?" This chapter tries to answer that question. "Things start to happen" after age 50—and especially after 65. Cancer, for example, becomes more and more frequent. Sudden death from a heart attack is a real possibility. In short, many older persons may be on the verge of a medical disaster, in spite of feeling fine.

The purpose of a complete physical is to look for conditions *before* they cause symptoms, when more can generally be done. A complete physical can also serve to search for signs of silent disease—including cancer and clogged arteries. In addition, it can identify risk factors and enable the doctor to educate the person appropriately, based upon what is found. This chapter reviews some of the periodic maneuvers which doctors perform, in addition to searching for cancer (which was covered in Chapter 3) and aside from immunizations (which are reviewed in Chapter 27).

AHA Recommendations for Periodic Examinations

The American Heart Association (AHA) recently revised its position on the use of periodic examinations. Exhibit 26–1 contains the AHA's latest recommendations.

The history-taking part of a complete history and physical exam might include questions from a "Health Survey Questionnaire" (provided in Appendix A). This is a comprehensive list of questions designed to make individuals more aware of any health problems

Exhibit 26–1   AHA's Recommendations on Periodic Examinations

---

A history and physical examination, including measurement of weight and blood pressure:
- every five years from age 20 to 60
- every $2\frac{1}{2}$ years from age 61 to 74
- every year after age 75

Blood pressure readings at $2\frac{1}{2}$ year intervals between the above exams from age 20 to 60

The following laboratory tests:
- fasting cholesterol and triglycerides by the same schedule as the history and physical examinations but optional after age 60, depending on previous results
- fasting blood sugar by the same schedule as the history and physical examinations but optional after age 75, depending on previous results

A baseline EKG at age 20, 40, and 60

A baseline chest x-ray at age 40

Source: American Heart Association.

they may have and assist them in bringing such problems to their doctor's attention. Most "yes" answers and some "no" answers might be cause for concern. In addition, a survey of one's diet is important. Note should be taken of the total calories, as well as the percentage of those calories that come from fats, and from saturated fats in particular. The amount of cholesterol and salt in the diet also should be noted. Other general dietary habits are important to know, such as who prepares one's food, how many meals a day one eats, and whether the diet is nutritionally balanced. One's exercise and physical activity habits should also be noted. More controversial, at this time, is the importance of a person's behavioral pattern—particularly whether one has life stresses and personality characteristics (such as the so-called "type A personality," one overly concerned with achievement, competition, and the pressures of time and responsibilities) which might increase the chances of a heart attack. Some authorities are convinced that certain persons will live longer by changing their personality type. Others remain skeptical.

The physical examination itself should include special attention to the heart and circulatory system. Examination of the blood pressure is discussed in Chapter 5. That part of the physical examination which is designed to search for cancer was discussed in Chapter 3.

Some of the laboratory tests noted in Exhibit 26–1 are discussed in more detail in Chapter 2. It should be mentioned that one's levels of triglycerides are far less important, in general, than one's cholesterol level. In addition to the tests mentioned above, less "cost-effective" but still useful screening tests—particularly in older persons—are a complete blood count, a complete urinalysis, a chemistry panel (a battery of tests—usually 18 to 23 in number— that measure certain body salts and liver enzymes, among other things), and thyroid function tests (to determine whether the thyroid gland might be over- or underactive). Some doctors believe that a blood test for syphilis should also be part of the data base.

Identifying Risk Factors

Identification of risk factors can be made after the above information is obtained. Of particular concern are those factors associated with heart attacks. These were discussed in greater detail in Chapter 2 and include cigarette smoking, high blood pressure, high cholesterol level, and being overweight. **For women, evaluation of one's risk for osteoporosis—and whether to take preventive measures—is best done at the very beginning of menopause** (see Chapter 9). Once risk factors are identified, your doctor can try to educate you about how to reduce those risks.

Education regarding accidents can be particularly useful. Accidents are the fourth leading cause of death for persons in general and the leading cause of death for persons under 45. After age 65 "accidents and adverse reactions" are the seventh leading cause of death. Most accidents occur in the home, followed by accidents in the workplace and motor vehicle accidents. However, motor vehicle accidents account for the most deaths, followed by falls, in a ratio of more than three to one. The most important counseling regarding accidents is for the doctor to encourage all persons to use seatbelts when riding in a motor vehicle. The next most important counseling measure for accidents is regarding safety measures designed to prevent falls in the home. These were reviewed in Chapter 8.

Problems Sometimes Overlooked in
Physical Examinations

Commonly neglected in evaluating the health of older persons are dental, vision, and hearing problems. Semiannual dental check-ups, especially, are valuable at all ages for those who still have teeth. While certain specific problems in these areas can be identified by a primary doctor at the time of a periodic exam, it is often necessary to see an appropriate specialist for treatment, as well as for certain diagnostic measures.

In older persons, reduced hearing often becomes a problem which generally ends up requiring referral for a hearing-aid evaluation, once correctable causes have been ruled out. Hearing and ear problems were discussed in Chapter 14. Primary care doctors can provide certain evaluations in the area of vision, such as distance and near-vision visual acuity, using wall eye charts and near-vision cards. The most important concern in the area of preventable blindness is **glaucoma**—a type of blindness associated with increased eye pressure, and usually highly treatable with regularly instilled eye drops. This disease is best detected by an ophthalmologist (an eye specialist). Glaucoma screening is ideally accomplished by a combination of tonometry (measurement of eye pressure), looking at the optic disc with special equipment, and visual field testing. Because glaucoma is somewhat uncommon, it is not "cost-effective" to screen for it. However—like all procedures which are not "cost-effective"—this is an area where one must judge for oneself where to "draw the line" in looking after one's health.

Glaucoma becomes increasingly common after age 40. It afflicts about one in every 125 to one in every 250 persons after age 40. However, it affects about one in every 25 persons after age 80. **All patients should have their eye pressure checked at age 40 and at least every two years thereafter, and more frequently if measurements are borderline normal or there is a positive family history of glaucoma.** Ophthalmologists generally measure the eye pressure and look at the optic disc during a routine complete eye exam. Visual field testing is typically performed when the pressures are elevated above normal and/or the optic discs appear to have glaucomatous changes. However, concerned persons should understand that visual field testing may be the best screening procedure for glaucoma, and that relying solely on a normal eye pressure may miss 30 to 50 percent of glaucoma cases.

Other causes of blindness that are treatable if caught early are much less common. Roughly 10 percent of cases of senile macular degeneration are treatable, but there is no known treatment for the other 90 percent (see Chapter 13). In addition, routine eye exams are useful for identifying and treating such common conditions as cataracts and for adjusting eye-glass prescriptions. How often one should have a routine eye exam depends in part on whether one wears glasses, or notes any difficulty with vision. Of course, near vision begins to decline in everyone after about age 40, and reading glasses may be needed for persons who never had to wear glasses previously. **A routine eye exam by an ophthalmologist every two to four years is a reasonable schedule for persons over 40 without specific eye problems.**

The Importance of Screening Procedures

This is not meant to be a complete listing of what might be offered in an "annual physical." Rather it is an attempt to outline some basic examinations that are generally available and widely considered useful by doctors. Other examinations might also be considered, depending on your age and sex, what is available in your community, how concerned you are about your health, and what you can afford. Medicare does not pay for screening exams of any sort, and most supplemental health insurance policies pay only a percentage of what Medicare allows; if Medicare pays nothing, they likewise pay zero. Thus, senior citizens must usually foot the entire cost of health screening exams themselves.

Although screening procedures and baseline examinations have traditionally been done at specially scheduled visits—such as during the so-called "annual physical"—there is no reason why patients should hesitate to ask for particular procedures or advice at the time of a problem-based visit. (Or—to look at things from the doctor's perspective—there is no reason why at least some parts of a screening exam—particularly important parts of the history taking, such as weight loss, appetite loss, and change in bowel habits—could not be also assessed at problem-based encounters.) On the other hand, there is no reason why certain screening procedures need necessarily be done if one does not feel comfortable with them, if the fear of certain parts of the exam would prevent one from having *any* kind of "physical" at all. Many older women, especially, feel uncomfortable having a Pap smear and rectal exam. They might feel reassured to learn that the Pap smear becomes less important after age 70, and the rectal exam only detects about 10 percent of colo-rectal cancers. In contrast, stopping cigarette smoking will do far more to increase longevity than a Pap smear and rectal exam. **However, mammography and stool testing for occult blood remain two of the most critical screening tests, and their importance in older persons cannot be overemphasized.** It is important to understand the overall perspective of which diseases strike in later life, and what measures provide the most potential benefit. Such an overview was provided in Chapter 1.

Chapter 27

IMMUNIZATIONS

Most people mistakenly think that immunizations are no longer necessary after childhood. This is not entirely true. Several immunizations are commonly given in adulthood—some of them increasingly important as one gets older.

Tetanus Immunization

Tetanus ("lockjaw") is fatal about half of the time, once it sets in. Although the classical case comes from the proverbial "stepping on a rusty nail," about a third of cases involve only minor wounds, or no awareness of having received *any* wound. Fortunately, this dreaded disease, thanks to immunization, is uncommon in this country; there are slightly less than a hundred cases each year. However, most cases occur in older persons—those over 60. Studies have shown that the majority of senior citizens are inadequately vaccinated. **Booster shots for tetanus should be carried out every 10 years to provide adequate immunity.** In cases of high-risk incidents, such as stepping on a rusty nail, it may be useful to get a booster earlier, if you have not had one within three years. However, adverse reactions to the vaccine tend to occur if one gets vaccinated too often. Vaccination more often than every three years is not recommended under any circumstances. Those who have never had the primary series of vaccinations in childhood need to have it as an adult.

Diphtheria Immunization

Diphtheria is considerably less of a danger to adults than tetanus. It is primarily a disease of the young and those who have never had any immunization against it. More than half the cases occur in persons less than 15 years of age. However, cases do occasionally occur, even in persons who are fully immunized against it. It is fatal in only about 10 percent of those who come down with it. Since there are only a few cases in this country each year, diphtheria immunization is less important than tetanus. Nevertheless, both should be maintained. Those who have never had the primary series of vaccinations in childhood need to have it as an adult. Like tetanus boosters, **diphtheria booster shots should be continued every ten years as an adult, if one has had the primary series in childhood.** Although tetanus vaccine is often combined with the diphtheria vaccine in a single shot, tetanus vaccine comes separately as well. Therefore, having had a tetanus booster within 10 years does not automatically mean that one also was immunized against diphtheria at that time.

Flu Shots

Most persons think of influenza ("the flu") as an illness which is more of a nuisance than something that can be fatal. Unfortunately, this is not always the case. People do die from influenza—especially older persons. When there are epidemics of flu, as many as 12 persons per 100,000 die from it. Many more than this died in the great flu epidemic of 1918. The category of influenza and pneumonia is the fifth leading cause of death in older persons.

Although older persons are more likely to suffer complications from the flu, **flu vaccine is recommended for *all* adults, regardless of age, if they are at high risk for pneumonia and bronchitis.** One way to know if you are at high risk is having a history of repeatedly getting pneumonia or bronchitis in winter. Asthmatics are generally at high risk, as are persons with "heart failure" (a term that generally is used by doctors to connote a chronic condition, rather than a fatal event). If you are not sure, ask your doctor. **Flu vaccine is also recommended for everyone over 65.** Although some authorities take the view that healthy persons do not need this vaccine, the view of the American College of Physicians is that, because of the possibility of unrecognized disease in older persons, even the so-called "healthy elderly" should be immunized.

Flu shots are best given between September and December. The best time of all is mid-October, in order to have adequate immunization through February and March, the reason being that the effectiveness of the vaccine begins to wane after about five months. You should not delay much past mid-October, however, since the flu season starts very soon afterward. It is all right to have a flu shot after that time; however, it takes about two weeks for immunity to build up. If flu breaks out in your community before this two-week period is over, you can get some protection by taking the drug amantadine (a prescription drug) in the meantime. Amantadine (Symmetrel) is not free of side effects. About 5 to 10 percent of adults who are given it suffer from irritability, trouble sleeping, lightheadedness, and difficulty concentrating. Older persons—especially those with failing kidneys—should receive lower than the usual dose.

You should not have a flu shot if you are allergic to eggs, since flu vaccine is made from eggs. If you have more of a reaction than a little swelling and redness of the arm after a flu shot, you should discuss with your doctor whether it is wise for you to have flu shots again in the future. While vaccines in general are quite safe, they are not 100 percent so.

Pneumococcal Vaccine

Contrary to popular belief, pneumococcal vaccine, often referred to as the "pneumonia shot," does not protect against all pneumonia—only against some 23 types of *pneumococcal* pneumonia. Studies indicate that the pneumococcus bacteria is the most prevalent and serious bacteria involved in respiratory infections. The pneumococcal vaccine offers some protection against more than 90 percent of the types of pneumococcal pneumonia which exist. Exactly how much protection is afforded has not been well studied. The best estimates are 70 to 80 percent protection in adults over age 60.

Those who choose to be vaccinated with pneumococcal vaccine should be aware that it generally should not be given more than once in a lifetime, because of a high incidence of side effects upon repeat vaccination. About half of persons who are vaccinated have local reactions of mild pain and swelling and redness at the site of the injection. About 1 to 5 percent get more severe reactions, such as fever, rash and joint pains. The benefits of pneumococcal vaccine last at least three to five years.

The pneumococcal vaccine is most valuable for persons who have had their spleens removed or who have sickle cell anemia. Although some authorities believe the vaccine is not needed except for persons in this group and the minority of persons who are at high risk for pneumonia, the American College of Physicians takes the view that—as in the case of the flu vaccine—**all persons over 65 should receive pneumococcal vaccination, including the so-called "healthy elderly," because of the possibility of unrecognized disease in older persons.** Because pneumococcal vaccine is given only once and because its benefits are thought to last from three to five years, just when a person should receive it should be carefully discussed with his or her doctor.

Unlike all other vaccinations and preventive health measures, pneumococcal vaccination is covered by Medicare. It can be given at the same time as the flu shot.

Part III

HEALTH-RELATED MATTERS

Chapter 28

PERSONAL DOCUMENTATION

It is important for older persons to understand a few basic facts about their own medical care. This is crucial when it comes to the names of drugs they take regularly, and any drugs to which they may be allergic or intolerant. The best way to avoid forgetting this information is to *write it down*. Best of all is to keep a copy of this information with you at all times. This advice becomes more important the older one gets, because older persons tend to take more medications and are more likely to have had reactions to drugs. If this information is not available, there is a greater chance that a doctor will prescribe the same drug that caused a bad reaction previously.

In the case of drug allergies, successive reactions tend to become progressively worse. Persons who may have had a bad reaction to penicillin, such as a very swollen tongue, may well end up having their airway blocked from a repeat dose, resulting in death. Patients who have had severe, life-threatening reactions to drugs often pass out within a few minutes of being given a shot of something to which they are allergic—usually penicillin. One woman who was allergic to penicillin but had forgotten this was quickly reminded of the fact when her tongue began to swell rapidly right after swallowing a penicillin tablet her dentist had prescribed. An ambulance was sent, and she was still conscious but with no recordable blood pressure by the time she reached the hospital. Although this woman survived the allergic reaction, numerous deaths occur in the United States each year from such causes. No doubt some of these deaths could have been avoided if the treating doctors had known the drugs to which the persons were allergic.

Another important reason for a doctor to know a patient's drug allergies is that many drugs are similar to each other. A history of a bad reaction to one drug will caution the doctor to avoid giving a different but related drug. But this is not the only reason to keep a written record of your drug allergies. You cannot rely on being able to recall the name of a drug to which you are allergic if it is prescribed again. Besides, there are so many brand names for various drugs, you might not be aware that you are being given the same drug under another name.

One fallacy on which many people rely for not bothering to carry this information with them is the belief that their personal doctor—who knows their case—will be available when they are sick. Unfortunately, that is not always the case. Sometimes people become ill while traveling far from home. Even at home, sick persons are often rushed by ambulance to the nearest hospital, and this may not be one where they have been previously. In such cases their past medical records will not be as readily available. This is especially true in cases of persons who are too ill to speak (and relate the name of their usual hospital). Too, their personal doctor may not be available quickly to provide information in time. (Doctors do sometimes take vacations.) Even when the doctor can be contacted promptly, the odds are against him or her actually being in the office at the time, and very few doctors keep copies of their patients' records elsewhere. (In the future, more doctors should be taking advantage of the computer revolution as a handy and relatively inexpensive way [currently about $4000] to keep at least certain crucial facts—such as patients' drug allergies—at home in a personal computer.*) Older people sometimes reassure themselves that such information will only be needed in the "unlikely event" of a medical emergency, but emergencies happen

---

*I recommend to interested doctors Apple's Macintosh Plus with internal drive, at least a 20 megabyte hard disc, Apple's Imagewriter (II or LQ) printer, Microsoft Word version 3.01 or greater for word processing (such as admitting history and physical exams), and Filemaker II as a data base both to generate periodic reminder letters for annual physicals and flu shots and to keep handy such crucial patient information as drug allergies and next-of-kin (as well as perhaps date of birth, Medicare number, and pharmacy). Much valuable time can be saved learning Word 3.01 by using the "Learn Word Series" (cassette-tape tutoring) from Personal Training Systems, P.O. Box 24431, San Jose, CA 95154 (Phone 408 559-8635).

to older people more often than they realize. It is better to be prepared.

For these reasons, it is most important for all persons—especially those over 65—to keep the following documents on their person at all times.

Wallet-Sized Cards of Basic Medical Information

A wallet-sized card providing basic medical information should be updated whenever there is significant new information or changes in your medication. Wallet-sized cards are available from the Medic Alert Foundation, and from the American Medical Association. The AMA's Emergency Medical Information Card is available by writing to:

American Medical Association
P.O. Box 10946
Chicago, Illinois 60610

The Medic Alert Foundation's address is given directly below.

Medical Identification Tags

A medical identification tag (necklace or bracelet), listing crucial information such as any drug allergies and the presence of important conditions such as diabetes should be worn at all times. (This can also be an excellent way—in the case of Medic Alert's tag—of routing access to a medical summary of one's condition where it can be obtained in an emergency by any doctor anywhere in the world.) There are at least two of these on the market. Best known is Medic Alert, which also has a 24-hour number that can be called to obtain any additional medical information you may wish to leave on file. For a Medic Alert enrollment form, write:

Medic Alert Foundation International
P.O. Box 1009
Turlock, CA 95381-1009

Medical identification bracelets and necklaces are also available from:

Body Guard
P.O. Box 747
Brigantine, NJ 08203

Wallet-Sized Baseline EKGs

A wallet-sized baseline EKG should be updated if you have a more recent EKG which has changed in any important way. This information is helpful to doctors in evaluating a suspected heart attack or heart rhythm disturbance. Without this information, it is more likely that you will be hospitalized unnecessarily. Once you have had an EKG made at your doctor's office, you can use a photocopy to make a wallet-sized EKG that you can carry on your person. Contact:

EKG Alertcard
1-800-EKG-5577

A Durable Power of Attorney for Health Care

A durable power of attorney for health care, a document described in more detail in the next chapter, allows you to delegate someone to make your health care decisions for you in case you are unable to do so yourself. It must be notarized or witnessed, and is usually valid for a period of up to seven years. A copy should be left with a responsible relative or friend. Your attorney should have a copy, as should your attorney-in-fact (the person designated to make your health care decisions for you if you become unable to do so yourself). You may obtain a copy by contacting:

California Medical Association
44 Gough St.
San Francisco, CA 94103

(415) 541-0900

Living Wills

A living will is a brief statement of your general desires regarding limits you wish placed on measures to prolong your life. It is discussed in more detail in the next chapter. You may obtain a wallet-sized copy by contacting:

Concern for Dying
250 W. 57 St.
New York, N.Y. 10107
(212) 246-6962

A contribution of $20 or more will get you a plastic-coated wallet card; smaller contributions will get a less-durable cardboard card.

Family Health Records

The American Medical Association has available a 12-page booklet entitled, "Family Health Record." It has sections for recording family history, immunizations, births, childhood diseases, health and accident insurance information, and other information. It also includes four detachable wallet-sized emergency medical information cards. The family health record should be brought to your physician at the time of any comprehensive exam and to the hospital at the time of any admission. It should be updated whenever there is new information. For details, write:

American Medical Association
P.O. Box 10946
Chicago, Illinois 60610

Personal Medication Record

A booklet called, "A Personal Medication Record," has been printed in the San Francisco Bay Area by the local health departments. It is a current, running record of all medications you take—both prescription and nonprescription. It is invaluable if you take more medications than you can easily keep track of by memory. You should bring it with you each time you go to the doctor. The booklet is available *free* to seniors 60 and older who live in the San Francisco Bay Area. It is available to others for 75¢. To get your copy, contact:

SRx, Seniors Medication Education Program
1183 Market Street, Room 204
San Francisco, CA 94102
(415) 558-3767

If you have never been hospitalized, you may wish to contact the medical records department of your hospital of choice and ask them to open a file on you. You can provide them with identifying information such as Medicare number, next of kin, etc. If you *have* been hospitalized previously at that hospital, you may wish to notify the medical records department of any important changes in your medical history or status. This is especially important should you develop an allergic reaction to any drug, or sign any legal document (such as a living will) which might affect your health care in the future.

Chapter 29

LEGAL PREPARATION

At the turn of the century, little thought was given to the question of what to do, in the way of medical care, for someone who was dying. That was because there was not much one *could* do. When one's time arrived, that was *it*.

Now that doctors can prolong life beyond the point where many would wish it, we often hear people saying things like, "I don't want to end up a vegetable—I'd rather die first." Such persons often demand of their relatives, "Don't ever use any tubes to keep me alive," "Don't ever use any machines to keep me going," or even, "Don't ever put me in a nursing home." Although the insistence against nursing home placement is often withdrawn once the difficulties of home care are faced, the desire not to have one's life prolonged by artificial means usually persists when a person is at the point of dying from natural causes at an advanced age.

Issues to Be Faced During a Terminal Illness

While we are in good health, the realities of what may lie ahead are still abstract. For most people, the issues eventually to be faced during a terminal illness turn out to be one or more of the following:

- To have the heart re-started, once it has stopped (called **cardiopulmonary resuscitation**);

251

- To have a breathing tube passed into the lungs (called **intubation**);
- To be "forced fed" from a tube passed to the stomach through the nose (called **tube feeding**);
- To have **intravenous fluids** used beyond a certain point;
- To have **antibiotics**—either by mouth or by some other route—used to treat pneumonia and other infections (such as urinary tract infections); and
- To be **re-hospitalized** after having been in and out of the hospital repeatedly while deteriorating with a terminal condition.

In practice, few people or their families opt for intubation or cardiopulmonary resuscitation; many ultimately decide to allow tube feedings, although many do not; most wish intravenous fluids used in the hospital setting, although there are occasional circumstances when even this modality is withheld; and those who have reached an advanced state of deterioration are often simply given morphine—rather than re-hospitalized—when pneumonia develops. Morphine is usually given by injection in the hospital or nursing home. At home, it can be given in a liquid form which is absorbed through the mouth, even for a person who is too weak to swallow. It can also be given by rectal suppository.

As if things are not difficult enough trying to decide which of these options is desired, matters are sometimes complicated by legal impediments, even when the family is clear about what they want for the patient. This may happen in cases of persons who never prepared a written statement of their desires. Terminally ill patients are often unable to speak for themselves. With this combination of events, the family sometimes prefers a course of treatment different from the one the doctor is pursuing.

Many people are not aware that there may be circumstances, such as the above, where the family cannot stop what measures are used to prolong the patient's life. If the patient remains at home, of course, things are different. No heroic measures will be used unless the family calls a doctor and has the patient transferred to a hospital. Once placed in the hospital, however, there may be circumstances where the wishes of the family may not matter. For example, the doctor may use life-sustaining measures even when the next-of-kin objects. A few years ago, this was the case at Brookside Hospital in San Pablo, California. A man who was comatose and dying of cancer was kept alive on a respirator because he had never indicated his desires while conscious. The son's objections went unheeded until he charged into the intensive care unit and ordered the nurse at gunpoint to unplug his father's respirator.

Not long before that, doctors at a hospital in southern California were charged with murder after unplugging the respirator of another terminally ill patient. Although the doctors were eventually exonerated, the fact that such charges could be filed in the first place underscores how dearly life is held in this country. Because of this, doctors are often reluctant to withdraw life-sustaining measures. In the absence of indications that a patient would not have wanted certain life-sustaining measures, doctors often feel it is their duty to provide them. When there are ethical dilemmas to be faced, hospital ethics committees, which are becoming increasingly available, can often assist the attending doctor in resolving the issues at hand. However, none of this can substitute for some kind of written document made by patients themselves when mentally competent and able to communicate, to indicate what they might wish in the way of medical care.

If preventive measures are important in the early detection of disease, they are doubly important when it comes to the legal aspects of treatment. For this reason, legal preparation is no less crucial than wearing an identification tag alerting doctors to any drug allergies you may have. Just as you may be unconscious when a doctor needs to know the drugs to which you may be allergic, so too might you be unconscious when a doctor needs to know your wishes regarding life-sustaining measures. In fact, the odds are far greater that you will be *unable* to speak when the latter information is germane.

Documents for Indicating One's Wishes Regarding Terminal Care

In "the good old days" (as some call them), when the doctor would more likely have known for decades not just the patient but the entire family, the legal aspects of medicine were less of a problem. The doctor more often knew just what to do. Nowadays—especially in urban areas and at large academic institutions—patients are sometimes cared for in a less personal manner. The treating doctor

may be only one member of a group practice or a large team, and
not long acquainted with the patient or the patient's family. In
such circumstances, it is especially important for patients to have
set down in writing their wishes regarding not just terminal care,
but measures that might apply even if they are *not* in a terminal
state. Three documents are particularly relevant: the living will,
the directive to physicians, and the durable power of attorney for
health care.

The Living Will

The **living will** is a brief statement requesting that the goal of any
medical treatment be limited to maintaining comfort in case one
has a terminal condition. The living will now carries the power of
law in at least 38 states* and the District of Columbia. Elsewhere
it offers no legal protection to the treating doctor who chooses to
respect the patient's wishes. For that reason, it may be best—in
states with no living will legislation—to have a document known as
a durable power of attorney for health care (described later in the
chapter). A complete living will declaration is provided in Exhibit
29–1.

A wallet-sized copy of the living will is available from Concern
for Dying. Concern for Dying also keeps a registry of living wills.
If your living will declaration is too lengthy to fit handily on a
wallet-sized card, a similarly sized card (provided by Concern for
Dying) can alert persons to the fact that your complete living will
declaration is on file. Concern for Dying is located at the following
address:

> Concern for Dying
> 250 W. 57 St.
> New York, N.Y. 10107
> (212) 246-6962

Because state laws vary, the required wording of a living will
declaration, as well as details regarding its execution (or revoca-
tion), will vary. For detailed information regarding specifics in each

---

*Alabama, Alaska, Arizona, Arkansas, California, Colorado, Connecticut, Delaware, Flor-
ida, Georgia, Hawaii, Idaho, Illinois, Indiana, Iowa, Kansas, Louisiana, Maine, Maryland,
Mississippi, Missouri, Montana, Nevada, New Hampshire, New Mexico, North Carolina,
Oklahoma, Oregon, South Carolina, Tennessee, Texas, Utah, Vermont, Virginia, Washington, West Virginia, Wisconsin, and Wyoming.

Exhibit 29–1   Living Will Declaration

LIVING WILL

To my Family, my Physician, my Lawyer, my Clergyman. To any Medical Facility in whose care I happen to be. To any individual who may become responsible for my health, welfare, or affairs.

Death is as much a reality as birth, growth, maturity, and old age—it is the one certainty of life. If the time comes when I, _____ (NAME), can no longer take part in decisions for my own future, let this statement stand as an expression of my wishes and directions while I am still of sound mind.

If a situation should arise when I am in a terminal state in which there is no reasonable expectation of my recovery from extreme physical or mental disability, I direct that I be allowed to die and not be kept alive by medications, artificial means, or "heroic" or extraordinary measures. I do, however, ask that medication be mercifully administered to me to alleviate suffering even though this may shorten my remaining life.

This statement is made after careful consideration and is in accordance with my strong convictions and beliefs. I want the wishes and directions here expressed carried out to the extent permitted by law. To the extent that the provisions and this Living Will are not legally enforceable, I hope that those to whom this Will is addressed will regard themselves as morally bound by them.

Optional specific provisions: [Here, one can add any personalized instructions desired.]

Dated _____   Signature _____

Witness _____   _____

_____

_____   Below signature, print or type full name and address of person

Witness _____   signing

_____

_____

Below signatures of witnesses, print or type their full names and addresses

Optional Notarization:

STATE OF: COUNTY OF:

"Sworn and subscribed to before me this ___day of _____, 19___ ."

_____
          Notary Public

          (SEAL)

Source: Phillip Williams, *The Living Will Source Book* (Oak Park, Illinois: The P. Gaines Company, 1986).

state, you may consult *The Living Will Source Book, With Forms,* by Phillip Williams (1986). The P. Gaines Company, P.O. Box 2253, Oak Park, IL 60303. ISBN 0-936284-22-6. Currently $14.95 plus $1.50 for shipping.

A way of expanding the usefulness of the living will to include conditions—such as Alzheimer's and other forms of dementia—when death is not imminent was suggested in a Letter to the Editor of the *Western Journal of Medicine* by Dr. W. A. Reynolds, associate professor of medicine at the University of Washington. Dr. Reynolds suggests signing an addendum to the living will in order to address this issue. The addendum he recommends is reproduced in Exhibit 29–2.

Dr. Reynolds' addendum, in brief, prohibits tube feedings, intravenous fluids, antibiotics, and transfer to a hospital for the purpose of prolonging life. However, one could still be transferred to a hospital for the purpose of repairing a broken bone, such as a hip. (Broken bones occur frequently in nursing home patients, and would be the most common reason for transferring such persons to an acute care hospital in the face of Dr. Reynolds' restrictions.)

Directive to Physicians

A document somewhat similar to the living will, but more detailed, is a **directive to physicians.** Like the living will, the directive to physicians specifies one's wishes in the way of health care when terminally ill. As with any other similar document, it must be legal in your state to provide your doctor the full protection of the law. (Without the full protection of the law, a doctor may be reluctant to withhold treatments—such as antibiotics and intravenous fluids—that you might not want but would customarily be given.)

The Durable Power of Attorney for Health Care

Because the living will and the directive to physicians are relevant only when death is imminent and relate only to measures which might sustain life, their applicability is less broad than that of a **durable power of attorney for health care (DPOAHC).** The latter has the potential to provide very specific guidance to doctors. There are many shades of grey in the practice of medicine, and every case is different. Prior to the occurrence of the actual situation, instructions can relate only to vague, fanciful possibili-

Exhibit 29–2 Addendum to a Living Will

The following are directions to my family, my physicians and the health care institutions where I may happen to be in the event that I am not able to make valid decisions about my future care.

If and when I am no longer mentally competent and there is little or no likelihood that I will regain mental competence as determined by my physicians, I not only request but demand that the following instructions for my care be followed:

1. If I am no longer able to eat in a normal manner, I do not wish to have my life prolonged by intravenous feedings and fluids, nor nasogastric, nor other gastric feedings. It is my wish to die if nutrition cannot be provided in the normal manner.

2. In the event of infections, including pneumonia or other serious infections, I do not want parenteral antibiotics or oral antibiotics which in any way could be interpreted as life-saving. If treatment will make nursing care easier, or if needed to prevent the spread of contagious infection, then appropriate treatment can be given. Urinary tract infections can be treated only by the oral route; I refuse any parenteral antibiotics. Topical treatments can be provided to improve nursing care.

I wish to emphasize that when I am no longer mentally competent, it is my wish to die in a normal course of events without benefit of medical intervention. If I am at home and can be taken care of there, I do not wish to be taken to a hospital for specific treatment, except in the case when nursing care is required that cannot be provided at home. If I am in a nursing home and become ill, I do not wish to be transferred to a hospital, the only exception being when it is impossible to provide the nursing care in the nursing home. Specifically, I refuse permission to be transferred to the hospital if the purpose is to prolong my life.

_____	_____
Date	Signed
_____	
Witness	
_____	
Witness	

Source: W. A. Reynolds, Correspondence in *The Western Journal of Medicine*, vol. 146, no. 4 (April 1987), p. 464. Reprinted by permission of the *Western Journal of Medicine*.

ties. By appointing an agent, the durable power of attorney for health care makes it possible for a decision to be based on the actual circumstances of the moment.

A power of attorney grants authority to another person—the "attorney-in-fact," or "agent"—to act on your behalf. You specify what powers to grant the agent and the time period during which these powers can be exercised. You can revoke the powers at any time. Ordinarily, the power of attorney ceases once you are no longer mentally competent. However, a *durable* power of attorney—if legal in your state—allows the powers of the agent to *continue*, even if you become incompetent. A lawyer may be helpful to you in filling out such a document, but is not generally needed.

California—considered a bellwether state in this area—legalized the durable power of attorney for health care in 1984. In this document, persons may either make their own statement concerning life-sustaining treatments and other health care matters, or choose from three prepared statements. The prepared statements of the DPOAHC provided by the California Medical Association (CMA) request, in brief, that (1) nothing be done to prolong one's life under *any* circumstances; (2) *everything possible* be done, regardless of the circumstances; or (3) everything possible be done *except* if in an irreversible coma, in which case *nothing* should be done. The document is valid for up to seven years. Exhibit 29–3 is a rudimentary version of a durable power of attorney.

Whether a similar document carries legal force in your own state is something you will need to determine by checking with your lawyer. You may obtain a copy of a durable power of attorney for health care from the CMA at the following address:

The California Medical Association
44 Gough St.
San Francisco, California 94103
(415) 541-0900

The CMA also provides with its DPOAHC a wallet card encaptioned, "Important Notice to Emergency Medical Personnel," on which one can list the names of one's agent and two alternates.

Concern for Dying (mentioned earlier in this chapter) has a related publication, "Appointing a Proxy for Health Care Decisions," available for $5.

Exhibit 29–3   Durable Power of Attorney for Health Care

I hereby designate _____to serve as my attorney-in-fact for the purpose of making medical treatment deci-sions. This power of attorney shall remain effective in the event that I become incompetent or otherwise unable to make such decisions for myself.

Dated _____   Signed _____

Witness _____   _____

_____   _____

_____   _____

_____

Witness _____

_____

_____

_____

(Below signatures of witnesses, print or type their full names and addresses.)

(Below signature, print or type full name and address of person signing.)

Source: Phillip Williams, *The Living Will Source Book* (Oak Park, Illinois: The P. Gaines Company, 1986).

Chapter 30

SUPPORT SYSTEMS

When one is suddenly faced with the problem of trying to help an older person whose health is failing but who does not need acute care hospitalization, it may seem there is nowhere to turn. However, that is not necessarily so. Although support services are rare in rural areas, in urban areas there are many, *if one knows where to look for them*. The problem is that social and health services—unlike federally funded Medicare—tend to be funded and administered on a local level, and this makes for much confusion when it comes to using them. In addition, these services are fragmented, often incomplete, and usually in flux because of frequently changing funding patterns.

An important aspect of these "ancillary" services is that it is sometimes necessary to get a doctor's authorization. This depends on whether funding for the program comes from the government. For example, a doctor's authorization is not needed to enter a nursing home, provided one is prepared to pay privately. But, for those who cannot afford to pay the considerable monthly fee or who are on welfare, the governmental body that does pay it— generally the state—requires a doctor's certification that the care is medically necessary. Meals on Wheels, on the other hand, is not funded by the state or federal government and therefore does not require a doctor's authorization. Some of the things which Medicare will pay for with a doctor's certification are hospital beds, wheelchairs, and specially designed mechanical chairs which lift the person partially toward the standing position.

Board and Care Homes

Sometimes senior citizens who have been living alone need placement in a more supervised setting. Commonly, such persons have
undergone such deterioration in memory that they no longer
remember to take their medicines—for example, their pills for
high blood pressure or glaucoma drops for the eyes. In board and
care homes (technically termed "community care facilities" and
also called "residential care facilities"), persons are on hand 24
hours a day to supervise such important routines as taking pills
and administering eye drops. Meals are served, and such amenities
as bed making and house cleaning are provided. Board and care
homes are licensed by the state, generally by the department of
social services, which can provide a list of facilities in your area.
Many facilities are also listed in the Yellow Pages under "Homes."
In general, board and care homes require that the resident be
independently ambulatory—at least with a cane—so as to be able
to leave the facility without help in case of a fire or other emergency. Needing a walker oversteps the bounds for which most
facilities are licensed. Nor will most board and care homes accept
patients who are incontinent. However, a small minority of such
facilities *are* licensed for persons who are incontinent, or who are
wheelchair- or in some cases even bed-bound.

The following important concerns should be investigated when
contemplating placement in a board and care home:

- Whether the person will have a private room and bath, or
  must share;
- Whether the room will be furnished;
- What activities are provided for the residents;
- What the food is like, and whether special diets can be
  provided when needed (e.g., for diabetics or persons who
  need to restrict salt);
- Whether the location is convenient to transportation and
  shopping areas.

Somewhere between the category of board and care homes and
nursing homes are continuing care communities, which provide a
comprehensive array of services beyond room and board. For more
information on such communities, write:

The American Association of Homes for the Aged
1050 17th St., NW
Washington, DC 20036

Nursing Homes

When patients require heavy care or begin to get bedsores, there
is generally no choice but to place them in a nursing home.
However, you should be prepared for a shock if you expect (as 41
percent of retirees mistakenly do) that Medicare or private insurance will pay for such care. In fact, only about 1 percent of patients
in nursing homes qualify for Medicare reimbursement; and most
private insurers pay only a portion of what Medicare allows.
Despite the *intensity* of care required, the vast majority of patients
in nursing homes are considered by Medicare to require only
"custodial care"—care which a family member could be taught
how to provide. Custodial care does not qualify for Medicare
reimbursement. Medicare only pays for what it terms "skilled
nursing care." An example of what Medicare calls skilled nursing
care is the administration of injections several times daily or
intravenous fluids. Other kinds of skilled nursing care which
qualify for Medicare reimbursement typically follow surgery. Examples are surgical wound treatments every 8 hours or physical
therapy twice a day after hip surgery.

A guide to private insurance policies for nursing home care is
provided in the May 1988 issue of *Consumer Reports* magazine,
"Who Can Afford a Nursing Home?" on pp. 300–311. (For subscription or other information, see Chapter 31.) Be advised that
the current state of affairs is bleak. To quote *Consumer's Reports*,

> We'd like to report that private insurance policies can meet the
> increasingly urgent need for long-term care coverage at a moderate
> cost. But many of the insurance policies we looked at were very
> expensive, severely limited in their coverage, or both.

Legislation to add long-term care benefits to the Medicare program
is now before Congress.

Your state government (department of health services) may have
booklets on how to choose a nursing home. In addition, here are
some other sources:

"How to Select a Nursing Home," available for $4.75 from:

Consumer Information Center
Department 152-M
Pueblo, CO 81009

A free guide to selecting a nursing home is available from:

Nursing Home Information Service
National Council of Senior Citizens
National Senior Citizens Education and Research Center, Inc.
925 15th St., NW
Washington, DC 20005
(202) 347-8800

A listing of nursing homes in your area can be obtained from a number of sources:

- The Yellow Pages of your phone book
- The social services department of your local hospital
- Your city or county health department
- Your state health department
- The senior information and referral service of your area's agency on aging

In choosing a nursing home, you may wish to consider the opinions of:

- Your clergyman
- Your doctor
- People you already know
- The residents of the home themselves and their families

Home Care

Because Medicare rarely pays for nursing home care, and never pays for care in a board and care facility, it is important to take advantage of support services that can assist older persons to maintain themselves at home. The problem is knowing just where to find such services. Here are some places to call:

- *Local Hospitals*. The social services or discharge planning department of your local hospital will have a list of local home care agencies. You do not have to be a patient to get the list.

- *Social Services Agencies*. These are charitable organizations sponsored by community or religious groups. They usually have special departments that deal with helping the aged.
- *Government Agencies*. Many city or county governments have senior information and referral services, which can put you in touch with various support services. They are administered by the department of public health.
- *Visiting Nurses*. There are two types of organizations here— government and private. *Public health nurses*, funded by city or county governments (at district health centers of the department of public health), can visit the patient in the home to perform an assessment and make needed referrals. *Private visiting nurse agencies* can also make home visits. Some home care benefits are paid for by Medicare; these are typically for persons who have just been discharged from a hospital. Some visiting nurse agencies are certified by Medicare; others are not. It is important to use one that is Medicare-certified in the case of services for which Medicare will pay. Even if Medicare *might* reimburse for a service, you will never receive that reimbursement if the service is not provided through a Medicare-certified agency.
- *Employment Services*. In addition to the above, a variety of home care agencies can provide workers, such as attendants, nurses aides, nursing assistants, live-in companions, occupational therapists, physical therapists, speech therapists, chore workers, LVNs and RNs, who can come to the home.

Many of the above are listed in the Yellow Pages under "Nurses and Nurses Registries."

Many churches and civic organizations have senior citizen groups. Other seniors groups are sponsored by state governments or the Salvation Army.

National Agencies

Many national agencies provide services especially geared toward older persons. The following is a fairly extensive listing of the most well known:

Alcoholics Anonymous
P.O. Box 459
Grand Central Station
New York, NY 10017

Alzheimer's Disease Society
32 Broadway
New York, NY 10004
(212) 425-1090

Alzheimer's Disease and Related
    Disorders Association
70 East Lake Street, Suite 600
Chicago, IL 60601
1-800-621-0379
[in Illinois, 1-800-572-6037]

American Association for the
    Education and Rehabilitation of
    the Blind and Visually Impaired
206 North Washington Street
Alexandria, VA 22314
(703) 548-1884

American Association of Geriatric
    Psychiatry
505 North Lake Shore Drive,
    Suite 1706
Chicago, IL 60611
(312) 329-0325

American Association of Retired
    Persons
1909 K Street N.W.
Washington, DC 20049
(202) 872-4700

American Cancer Society
90 Park Avenue
New York, NY 10016
1-800-ACS-2345

American Council for the Blind
501 North Douglas Avenue
Oklahoma City, OK 73106
1-800-424-8666

American Diabetes Association
1660 Duke St.
P.O. Box 25757
Alexandria, VA 22314
1-800-232-3472

American Foundation for the Blind
15 West 16th Street
New York, NY 10011
1-800-AFB-LIND

American Heart Association
7320 Greenville Avenue
Dallas, Texas 75231
(214) 750-5300
1-800-527-6941

American Jewish Congress
15 E. 84 Street
New York, NY 10028
(212) 879-4500

American Lung Association
1740 Broadway
New York, NY 10019
(212) 315-8700

American Optometric Association
243 North Lindbergh Boulevard
St. Louis, MO 63141
(314) 991-4100

American Parkinson Disease
    Association
116 John St.
New York, NY 10038
1-800-223-APDA
[in New York State, 1-800-732-
    9550]

American Society on Aging
833 Market St.
San Francisco, CA 94103
(415) 543-2617

American Speech-Language-
Hearing Association
10801 Rockville Pike
Rockville, MD 20852
(301) 897-5700

American Red Cross
17th and D Streets, N.W.
Washington, DC
(202) 737-8300

Arthritis Foundation
National Office
1314 Spring Street, N.W.
Atlanta, GA 30309
(404) 872-7100

Books on Tape
P.O. Box 7900
Newport Beach, CA 92660
1-800-626-3333

Catholic Charities, USA
1319 F St., N.W.
Washington, DC 20004
(202) 639-8400

Cancer Information Service
1-800-4-CANCER
1-800-422-6237

Gerontological Society
1411 K Street, N.W., Suite 300
Washington, DC 20005
(202) 393-1411

National Association for Homecare
519 C Street, N.E.
Washington, DC 20002
(202) 547-7424

National Association for the
Visually Handicapped
22 West 21st Street, 6th Floor
New York, NY 10010
(212) 889-3141

National Clearinghouse for Alcohol
Information
Box 2345
Rockville, MD 20852
(301) 468-2600

National Council of Churches
475 Riverside Drive
New York, NY 10115
(212) 870-2200

National Council on the Aging
650 South Spring Street, Suite 721
Los Angeles, CA 90014
(213) 622-6151

National Council on Alcoholism,
Inc.
733 Third Avenue
New York, NY 10017
(212) 206-6770

National Diabetes Information
Clearing House
Box NDIC
Bethesda, MD 20205
(301) 496-4000

National Federation of the Blind
1800 Johnson St.
Baltimore, MD 21230
(301) 659-9314

National Hospice Foundation &
Home Care
519 C Street, N.E.
Washington, DC 20002
(202) 547-6586

National Library Service for the
Blind and Physically
Handicapped
Library of Congress
1291 Taylor Street, N.W.
Washington, DC 20542
(202) 287-5100

National Retinitis Pigmentosa
  Foundation
8331 Mindale Circle
Baltimore, MD 21207
(301) 225-9400

National Self-Help Clearinghouse
33 W. 42nd Street, Room 1206A
New York, NY 10036
(212) 840-1259

National Kidney Foundation
2 Park Avenue
New York, NY 10016
(212) 889-2210

National Mental Health Association
1021 Prince St.
Alexandria, VA 22314-2932
(703) 684-7722

National Society to Prevent
  Blindness
500 East Remington Road
Schaumburg, IL 60173
1-800-221-3004

Rehabilitative Services
  Administration
Office for the Blind & Visually
  Impaired
330 C Street, S.W.
Washington, DC 20201
(202) 245-0918

Local Agencies

Many of the foregoing national agencies have local chapters or units. In addition, there are many agencies or services on the state and local level which are similar throughout the country, including the following:

Commission on the Aging (in most large cities)
County Dental Society
County Medical Society
Friendship Line for the Elderly
Hearing and Speech Center (you can contact the American Speech-Language-Hearing Association, listed above, to find out the number of your local Hearing and Speech Center)
Lighthouse for the Blind (in most major cities)
Mental Health Association of (your city)
Mental Health Information and Referral Service
Salvation Army (in your city)
Smoking Education (see American Lung Association)
State Bar Association (for legal referral)
State Commission for the Blind and Visually Impaired
State Department of Education
State Department of Rehabilitation
State Medical Association

State Podiatric Association

Suicide Prevention Hotline (check under "Suicide," in the phone book)

Other Local Agencies and Services

Besides the foregoing, there are a variety of other services and agencies on the local level that are organized in a more fragmented way. Many of them provide services to elders who are homebound or who have other special problems:

Adult Day Health Centers. A variety of organizations, such as visiting nurse associations, hospitals, charitable organizations, and city and county governments, sponsor adult day health centers. They provide rehabilitative services, social services, hot noon meals, nutritional counseling, transportation to and from the center, and nursing and personal care. They also provide case managers who assess persons as to their functional impairments, both physical and mental. They are useful for assisting persons to continue to take care of themselves so they can remain in the community and avoid nursing home placement.

Lifeline Emergency System. Devices such as necklaces are now available which older persons can wear to summon an ambulance in case they are unable to get to a phone. Many hospitals have programs which work in conjunction with these devices. For example, the hospital may expect a person to "check in" by telephone once daily before 10 P.M. to confirm that he or she is all right. Some devices are programmed to call the 911 emergency assistance number (if it exists in your area) or the local police department. A local hospital which has such a system may be able to refer you to a nearby company that can sell and install such a device on your phone. Or, you can look in the Yellow Pages under "Security Control Equipment & Systems" or "Telephone Equipment & Systems—Dealers." Or, you can contact one of the companies listed under that product in the American Association of Retired Persons' publication, *The Gadget Book*, reviewed in the next chapter.

Senior Citizens' Service Organizations. Many of the organizations referred to elsewhere in this chapter are listed in the Yellow

Pages under the heading, "Senior Citizens' Service Organizations." Some of the services listed here are:

- Adult Day Health Centers
- Alcoholism Information and Treatment Centers for the Elderly
- Charter Bus Tours for Senior Groups
- Church and Religious Groups who offer programs for the Elderly
- Friendship Line for the Elderly
- Legal Assistance to the Elderly
- Medical Claims Services (assist you to fill out health insurance forms)
- Network of Volunteers who serve the Elderly
- Senior Centers
- Senior Citizens Information and Referral Service
- Senior Escort Programs
- Social Workers who specialize in Case Management for the Elderly

Social Service Organizations.   A number of social service organizations (not listed under the previous heading) which provide services to seniors are listed under the heading "Social Service Organizations" in the Yellow Pages. Some examples are:

- Blind, National Federation of the (local offices)
- Catholic Social Service
  —Aging Services
  —Hearing Impaired Program
- Family Service Agency Geriatric Day Treatment
- Meals on Wheels
- National Association for the Visually Handicapped
- Retired Senior Volunteer Program
- YMCA
- YWCA
  —Senior Citizen Apartments

Geriatric Services.   There may be several listings in the White Pages under the heading "Geriatric Services" for various services for elders.

In-Home Support Services.   The Senior Information and Referral Service of your local department of public health can provide you with a list of agencies that can provide services in the home to help frail older adults who become homebound for a short or long period of time. Several types of support service personnel can assist in the home, depending on the particular needs of the individual. The following are examples of some of these professionals:

- *Registered nurse (RN)*. A professional nurse who is licensed by the state Board of Registered Nurses; the RN can provide "skilled nursing care," which includes providing treatment prescribed by a physician and giving medications, as well as providing education to patients and their families.
- *Licensed vocation nurse (LVN)*. A practical nurse without the training and experience of a registered nurse.
- *Home health aide*. Provides help with personal hygiene, such as bathing, dressing and toileting, and with meal preparation, handling medical equipment, and other activities of daily living.
- *Homemaker*. Helps the patient and family with household tasks such as cleaning, laundry, and housekeeping.
- *Medical social worker*. Provides counseling and support, is knowledgeable about resources in the community, and can assist in obtaining placement at a higher level of care, such as boarding or nursing home.
- *Registered dietician*. Provides counseling for special diets, such as elders who need to gain or lose weight, or who have special dietary restrictions, such as for diabetes, hypertension, heart failure, or gout.
- *Physical therapist*. Assists the individual with mobility problems through exercise programs to improve strength, mobility, and coordination; or by the use of heat, cold, or other treatments to help control pain and stiffness of the muscles, bones, and joints.
- *Occupational therapist*. Assists persons with handicaps or disabilities to function more independently in the activities of daily living such as eating, dressing, and toileting.
- *Speech therapist*. Provides instruction and treatment to patients with speech and language problems—typically those who have Parkinson's disease or who have had a stroke which affected speech and language abilities.

Before hiring someone to come into the home, you should seek out answers to questions such as the following:

- Does the person have references?
- Are a minimum number of hours required?
- How much does the agency charge per hour?
- Is the person bonded and insured by the agency?
- Is the person supervised by the agency?
- Does the agency provide for a backup person in case the original person becomes ill or fails to show up?
- Is the service paid for by Medicare or by welfare?
- How do you terminate the service once it is no longer needed, or if the worker is unsatisfactory?

If you are not sure just what services you need, the Senior Information and Referral Service can provide you with some names of persons—generally nurses or social workers—who can act as case managers.

Geriatric Mental Health Services

Most city and county governments provide psychiatric evaluation services, including counseling of individuals and families, day treatment care, and supportive services.

Resource Guides

Some city and county governments publish resource guides of local services for seniors in general, or for the homebound elderly. They are published by the city or county department of public health, Office of Senior Information Referral and Health Promotion.

Miscellaneous Community Services for Seniors

Many communities provide a variety of other special services for seniors, including the following.

Banking. Many banks have a "bank by mail" program. There is a "direct deposit" program by which you can have your social security check deposited directly to your bank account each month, rather than first sent to your home. You can withdraw cash from your account by sending a personal collector with a note and your signature. However, it is best to contact the bank manager beforehand. For those who need help with financial management, organizations in your area with names such as Support Services for

Elders can provide such assistance for a moderate fee. They would be listed under "Social Service Organizations" in the Yellow Pages.

Cleaners. When sending out your garments to be cleaned or laundered, be sure to first check the pockets and remove all items. You should make a list of all the items being sent, and refer back to it when they are returned to be sure nothing is missing. Be sure to alert the cleaner if the garment has a belt or other accessory, and point out any spots which need special treatment. Many cleaners will pick up and deliver for an extra fee.

Dental Programs. In some areas dentists will accept reduced fees for seniors who have limited means but do not have welfare or dental insurance. You should check with your local dental society.

Fire Department Invalid Sticker Program. It is important for you to alert the local fire department if you are homebound and incapacitated and might have difficulty getting out of your building or home in case of fire. The fire department will send someone to your home to review safety regulations with you and alert the fire station nearest you of your predicament. This could be a lifesaving measure in the event of a fire or other emergency situation in your building. You should call the Management Service Office of the fire department and inquire about the Invalid Sticker Program.

Financial Help with Utilities. The local gas and electric company may have special programs for the elderly needy, including those who have extra energy needs to operate life-support machines or other medical equipment. You should speak with a customer assistance representative.

Grocery Delivery. Many groceries and markets provide phone ordering and delivery services to nearby customers, often at no extra charge with a minimum purchase. You should start by checking with your usual grocery store.

Hearing Services. Many hearing centers will perform services in the home, including hearing testing, fitting of hearing aids, repairs, and battery changes. If there is a local hearing society, you should inquire about loans for hearing aids.

Home Maintenance and Repairs. For small home repairs you should look in the Yellow Pages under "Home Repairs and Maintenance," or look at ads in your local newspaper, or call the senior information and referral office for inexpensive handy persons. For larger jobs which require contractors, contact your local Better Business Bureau for their free book, *Consumer Resource Book and Membership Roster*.

To register complaints about a business, you should call the Better Business Bureau and/or the Contractor's State License Board of the state department of consumer affairs.

In some areas the local gas and electric company sponsors special programs to provide low-income seniors over 60 with free weatherization. It may be called, "Free Weatherization H.E.L.P. Program."

Persons of low to moderate income who own their own homes may be able to get an interest-free loan to correct code violations. You should inquire with the local department of public works to see if there is such a fund in your area.

Legal Assistance. The local Bar Association will usually provide referrals to persons of any age. In some areas there may be an organization that specializes in providing legal assistance to the elderly. You should look in the Yellow Pages under "Social Services" or "Senior Citizen Services." The American Jewish Congress, which has branch offices in many communities, provides free legal counseling for any senior citizen who qualifies financially.

Library Services. Some libraries have volunteers who will pick up and deliver books to homebound seniors. Some libraries have a Blind and Print Handicapped Library, which may be able to accept phone orders and mail the books to persons with such handicaps. Some libraries have videotapes for the deaf. Many libraries have mobile branches which travel to underserved or economically disadvantaged areas on a weekly or monthly basis.

Medical Supplies and Equipment. Companies which provide products to enhance the comfort and safety of homebound persons are listed in the Yellow Pages under "Hospital Equipment and Supplies." The supplier can furnish you with information regarding coverage by government programs.

Generic Drugs. If you wish to save money, one way is to ask your doctor to allow you to have a generic substitute for the prescription drugs you take. In most cases, there is no significant difference in the quality, but the savings can be considerable. Even more of a savings can be made by ordering your drugs in larger quantity (usually at least 90 days' worth at a time) through mail order companies, such as those listed in Exhibit 31–1 in the next chapter.

If you need to have your medications delivered, be sure to have the prescription phoned into a pharmacy which will make home deliveries. You also might wish to do comparison shopping among pharmacies before it is time to refill your prescription. Often there is a wide difference in price for the same drug at different pharmacies.

When you are calling your doctor to ask for a refill of a drug, have the name and phone number of the pharmacy ready.

Postal Services for the Homebound. The post office will provide stamps by mail for a small charge. Call your main post office and ask for the stamp by mail form.

Prepared Meals. Many cities have Meals on Wheels programs, which deliver nutritious meals to seniors who are unable to prepare adequate meals for themselves. Some senior centers also provide this kind of service to seniors in their areas. A number of restaurants also will deliver meals within certain areas. You can check the Yellow Pages for restaurants that advertise delivery service.

Senior Escort Services. Some cities have volunteer escort services that will provide someone to accompany seniors who live in dangerous areas to doctor's appointments, or to go shopping, or even to take a walk.

Tax Assistance. The Internal Revenue Service provides tax assistance free of charge to seniors. There are also private businesses that will perform tax assistance in the home. They can be found in the Yellow Pages.

Transportation Services. The American Cancer Society's local branches in many cities will provide free transportation for cancer patients to radiation and chemotherapy appointments. Some hospitals provide free transportation for nonemergency admissions and ambulatory (come-and-go) surgery. Some hospital clinics and most welfare programs provide taxi vouchers for doctors' appointments. Similar services are available for "ambuvan" transportation, which provides transportation via special vehicles equipped to transport persons in wheelchairs.

Veterinary Services. Some veterinarians will make house calls for pets with minor problems. Some do not charge extra, and some give seniors a discount.

Voting. Seniors who find themselves temporarily homebound can generally vote in an election by writing a month in advance to the registrar of voters, city hall, to request an absentee ballot. Be sure to include your name, address, phone number, and signature. If you are permanently homebound, you can request a special handicapped form from the registrar of voters. You will then be sent an absentee ballot automatically at every election.

Chapter 31

BECOMING INFORMED

A considerable amount of information on health and related topics is available to senior citizens, and much of it is free. This chapter lists pamphlets and booklets, newsletters, books, health libraries, hotlines, gadgets, and other health-related services for senior citizens.

Pamphlets and Booklets Listed by Topic

Many organizations offer pamphlets and booklets either free (for single copies) or at low cost. When sending for free literature, you should always enclose a self-addressed, stamped, business-size (no. 10) envelope. The listings below are presented first by topic, then by source.

Breast Cancer

The following booklets are available free from the American Cancer Society—either the national headquarters or your local unit (listed in the White Pages). For the address and phone number of the national headquarters, please see the listing in Chapter 30.

- "How to Examine Your Breasts"
- "Mammography—Saving More Lives"
- "Facts on Breast Cancer"
- "Good News That May Save Your Life"

Another source of free materials on breast cancer is the Breast Cancer Education Program. It offers the following pamphlets:

- "Breast Exams: What You Should Know"
- "Questions and Answers About Breast Lumps"
- "Breast Biopsy: What You Should Know"

These booklets can be obtained by writing to:

Breast Cancer Education Program
Office of Cancer Communications
National Cancer Institute
Building 31, Room 10A18
Bethesda, MD 20205

An excellent booklet, "A Step-by-Step Guide to Breast Self-Examination," was developed by Carol Case., R.N., M.Ed., Director of the Breast Cancer Education Program of the National Cancer Institute, in conjunction with *Primary Care and Cancer Magazine*, a professional journal. It is available for $1.00 and return postage from:

BSE Guide
P.O. Box 86
Williston Park, NY 11596

Another booklet called, "Mammography: A Patient's Guide to Breast x-ray Examination," is available free from:

The American College of Radiology
1891 Preston White Drive
Reston, VA 22091

The pamphlet, "Breast Cancer: Your Best Protection . . ." is available from:

National Cancer Foundation
Cancer Care, Inc.
1180 Avenue of the Americas
New York, NY 10036

Bowel Cancer

The following pamphlets on bowel cancer are available free from the American Cancer Society:

- "Colorectal Cancer: Go for Early Detection"
- "Facts on Colorectal Cancer"

Other Cancers

The following pamphlets on cancer are available free from the American Cancer Society:

- "Facts on Ovarian Cancer"
- "Facts on Prostate Cancer"
- "Facts on Bladder Cancer"
- "Facts on Lung Cancer"
- "Facts on Uterine Cancer"
- "Stay Healthy: Learn About Uterine Cancer"
- "Endometrial Cancer"
- "For Men Only: What You Should Know About Prostate Cancer"
- "Nutrition and Cancer: Cause and Prevention"
- "50 Most Asked Questions" (about smoking and health)

Smoking

The following pamphlets are available free from the American Cancer Society:

- "Quitter's Guide"
- "The Decision Is Yours" (to stop smoking)
- "Dangers of Smoking: Benefits of Quitting"

The following booklets are available from the American Lung Association (address listed on page 266):

- "Freedom from Smoking in 20 Days"
- "A Lifetime of Freedom from Smoking" (to read after having quit)

The following booklets are available from the American Heart Association (local unit listed in the White Pages, or see page 266 for listing of the national office):

- "Smoking and Heart Disease"
- "Calling It Quits" (a self-help kit)

The National Cancer Institute has the following free booklets:

- "Clearing the Air: A Guide to Quitting Smoking"
- "The Quit for Good Kit"

They are available free from:

> Publications Orders
> Office of Cancer Communications
> National Cancer Institute
> National Institutes of Health, Bldg. 31, Room 10A18
> Bethesda, MD 20892

A quit-smoking kit, "The Stanford Quit Kit," has been developed by Stanford University. For information, write:

> Stanford Health Promotion Resource Center
> HRP Building, Room 113
> Stanford, CA 94305-5090

Heart Disease

Two important booklets on heart disease are available from the American Heart Association (your local chapter of the national office, listed on page 266):

- "Smoking and Heart Disease"
- "An Active Partnership for the Health of Your Heart"

The booklet, "How Doctors Diagnose Heart Disease," by the U.S. Department of Health and Human Services, Public Health Service, National Institutes of Health (NIH Publication No. 80-753, reprinted August 1980) is available from:

> Public Inquiries and Reports Branch
> Department RL
> National Heart, Lung, and Blood Institute
> Building 31, Room 4A21
> National Institutes of Health
> Bethesda, MD 20205

Also available from the above source is the booklet, "Facts About Blood Cholesterol," Revised 1985, 3 pages, NIH Publication No. 85-2696.

"The Human Heart: A Living Pump" is an illustrated brochure which explains how the heart works. It is DHEW Publication No. (NIH)76-1058, and is for sale by:

Superintendent of Documents
U.S. Government Printing Office
Washington, DC 20402

High Blood Pressure

The High Blood Pressure Information Center has two very useful booklets. The first, "Questions About Weight, Salt, and High Blood Pressure" (1980, printed 1986, 12 pages. NIH Publication No. 86-1459), describes what is known about the relationship between dietary changes and high blood pressure. The second, "High Blood Pressure and What You Can Do About It" (1980, 32 pages, the Benjamin Publishing Company), describes the serious nature of high blood pressure, myths and facts about the disease, drugs used, and suggestions for staying with therapy. Both booklets can be obtained by contacting:

High Blood Pressure Information Center
120/80 National Institutes of Health
Bethesda MD 20892
(301) 496-1809

Obesity

The booklet, "Obesity and Your Health," is available from:

American College of Obstetricians and Gynecologists
600 Maryland Avenue, S.W., Suite 300 East
Washington, MD 20024-2588

Osteoporosis

The National Dairy Council has the following three booklets on osteoporosis:

- "Calcium: You Never Outgrow Your Need For It"
- "Are You at Risk for Bone Disease?"
- "The All-American Guide to Calcium-Rich Foods"

They are available free from:

National Dairy Council
6300 North River Rd.
Rosemont, IL 60018

The booklet, "Osteoporosis," is available from:

American Academy of Orthopedic Surgeons
P.O. Box 618
Park Ridge, IL 60068

Nutrition

The useful booklet, "Food 3," is available from:

American Dietetic Association
P.O. Box 91403
Chicago, IL 60693

The American Heart Association (address listed on page 266) offers free single copies of the following titles:

- "Nutrition Labeling: Food Selection Hints for Fat-Controlled Meals," 10 pages, #50-040A
- "Recipes for Fat-Controlled Meals from the American Heart Association Cookbook," 1981, 36 pages, #50-020B
- "The Way to a Man's Heart: A Fat-Controlled, Low Cholesterol Meal Plan to Reduce the Risk of Heart Attack," 8 pages, #40-018A

Parkinson's Disease

The following booklets are available from the American Parkinson Disease Association (address listed on page 266):

- "Home Exercises for Patients with Parkinson's Disease"
- "Parkinson's Disease Handbook: A Guide for Patients and Their Families"
- "Speech Problems and Swallowing Problems in Parkinson's Disease"
- "Aids, Equipment and Suggestions: To Help the Patient with Parkinson's Disease in the Activities of Daily Living"

The booklet, "One Step at a Time: An Exercise Manual for the Parkinsonian Patient," is available free from:

The United Parkinson Foundation
360 W. Superior St.
Chicago, IL 60610
(312) 664-2344

Vision

The booklet, "Seeing Well as You Grow Older," is available from:

The American Academy of Ophthalmology
P.O. Box 7424
San Francisco, CA 94120-7424

For information about large-print books, contact:

Doubleday Large Print Home Library
1-800-343-4300, ext. 355

Taking Medications

The booklet, "Using Your Medicines Wisely: A Guide for the Elderly," is available free from:

Health Advisory Services Program Department
American Association of Retired Persons
1909 K Street, N.W.
Washington, DC 20049

Quackery

A booklet entitled, "Quackery and the Elderly," is available free from:

Food and Drug Administration
HFE-88
5600 Fishers Lane
Rockville, MD 20857

Saving Money/Health Insurance

"Saving Tips for Health" (financial advice on using your health care dollar prudently) is available free from:

Saving Tips for Seniors
United Seniors Consumer Cooperative
1334 G St., N.W.
Washington, DC 20005

"I Can't Believe I'm Not Covered . . . There Must Be Some Mistake!" is a pamphlet listing insurance companies which offer long-term care health insurance. It is available free from:

California Association of Health Facilities
1251 Beacon Blvd.
West Sacramento, CA 95691-3461
(916) 371-4700

Another useful booklet, "How to Use Private Health Insurance with Medicare," discusses how to get coverage for what Medicare does not pay. It is available from:

Health Insurance Association of America
1850 K Street, N.W.
Washington, DC 20006

Booklets with advice on purchasing health insurance can be obtained from your state Medical Association.

The American Medical Association offers two excellent brochures on the financial aspects of health care:

- "What You Can Do About Health Care Costs" (OP-397)
- "Let's Talk About Health Insurance" (OP-342).

These booklets can be obtained by contacting:

Book and Pamphlet Fulfillment
AMA
P.O. Box 10946
Chicago, IL 60610
(Credit card orders may be directed to the toll-free number, 1-800-621-8335.)

If you take more than one or two medications on a daily basis, it may be well worth your while to explore the savings to be gained by requesting generic drugs (with your doctor's approval), by comparison shopping at local pharmacies, and by ordering your medication in larger quantities—3 months' to a year's supply or more—from mail-order pharmacies. Anyone can order drugs by mail. However, in the case of some mail-order plans, you must first join an organization with which the plan is affiliated. In order to get your medications by mail you will need a doctor's prescription, typically for at least a 90-day supply. However, some pharmacies are willing to call your doctor for authorization. Exhibit 31–1 lists some mail-order pharmacies.

Support Services

There is a useful booklet, "A Home Away from Home: Consumer Information on Board and Care Homes," with a foreword by Congressman Claude Pepper. It is available free from:

Exhibit 31-1   Mail-Order Pharmacies That Serve the Public

	Phone
Retired Persons Pharmacy[1]	For the toll-free number of the pharmacy that serves your area, call either AARP headquarters in Washington, D.C. (202-872-4700) or the AARP membership office in Lakewood, CA (213-496-2277).
America's Pharmacy *P.O. Box 10490* *Des Moines, IA 50306*	800-247-1003
Action Mail Order Drug *P.O. Box 787* *Waterville, ME 04901*	207-873-6226
National Pharmacies[2] *P.O. Box 1000* *Elmwood Park, NJ 07407*	800-631-7780
Nationwide Prescription *C.S. 2080* *Valley Stream, NY 11582*	800-252-1122
Walgreens *519 West Lone Cactus* *Phoenix, AZ 85027*	800-345-1985
Family Pharmaceuticals *P.O. Box 1288* *Mt. Pleasant, SC 29464*	800-922-3444
Prescription Delivery Systems *49 South York Rd.* *Hatboro, PA 19040*	800-441-8976

[1]Open to the general public, but discounts available to American Association of Retired Persons (AARP) members, who must be at least 50 years old and pay $5 per year. (AARP, Membership Information, 3200 E. Carson St., Lakewood, CA 90712. Telephone 213-496-2277.)

[2]Nonfunded participation through National Council of Senior Citizens. Membership in NCSC, which costs $12 per year ($16 per year for couples), has no age restrictions and is open to the general public. (NCSC, 925 15th St. N.W., Washington, D.C. 20005. Telephone 202-347-8800.)

Source: "Prescription Drugs," *Consumer's Checkbook Magazine* (Washington, D.C., 1987).

Tina McPherson
AARP
1909 K Street, N.W.
Washington, DC 20049

The National Support Center for Families of the Aging has a seminar program called, "Help for Families of the Aging," consisting of three cassette tapes and a workbook ($17.95). The seminar

covers ways of avoiding caregivers' burnout and methods of mean-
ingful communication with the elderly. The NSCFA also offers a
booklet, "Families and Aging: Resources for Individuals and
Groups" ($ 4.75), which lists books and periodicals about caregiv-
ing. For information, write:

> The National Support Center for Families of the Aging
> P.O. Box 245
> Swarthmore, PA 19081
> (215) 544-5933

Miscellaneous Topics

The pamphlet, "Aging and Digestion," is available from:

> The National Institute on Aging
> Information Center
> 2209 Distribution Circle
> Silver Spring, MD 20910

The National Institute on Aging also has many other publications.
You may wish to request a publication list.

Pamphlets and Booklets Listed by Source

There are several particularly rich sources of free and low-cost
information for senior citizens. Here we recommend publications
from the federal government, *Consumer Reports*, the American
Association of Retired Persons, and the Metropolitan Life Insurance Company.

U.S. Government Consumer Information Catalogue

To get any of the booklets below, or to request a catalogue, write
to:

> R. Woods
> Consumer Information Center-X
> P.O. Box 100
> Pueblo, CO 81002

Some booklets are free, and others are available at nominal cost
(approximate price listed). There is a $1.00 charge for ordering two

or more free booklets. The catalogue itself is free. The following booklets are available:

- "Guide to Health Insurance for People with Medicare." Free.
- "For Treating Arthritis, Start with Aspirin." Free.
- "Generic Drugs: How Good Are They?" Free.
- "Some Things You Should Know About Prescription Drugs." Free.
- "Fitness Fundamentals." Approx. $1.00.
- "Walking for Exercise and Pleasure." Approx. $1.00.
- "Calories and Weight." Approx. $2.25.
- "Cancer Prevention: Good News, Better News, Best News." Free.
- "Clearing the Air: A Guide to Quitting Smoking." Free.
- "The Dental Plaque Battle Is Endless, But Worth It." Free.
- "Everything Doesn't Cause Cancer." Free.
- "Insomnia." Free.
- "Protect Your Lifeline—Fight High Blood Pressure." Approx. $2.00.
- "Stroke." Approx. $1.75.
- "Ulcers." Free.
- "Varicose Veins." Approx. $1.00.
- "A Consumer's Guide to Mental Health Services." Free.
- "Plain Talk About Mutual Help Groups." Free.
- "Plain Talk About Physical Fitness and Mental Health." Free.
- "Diet and the Elderly." Free.
- "Nutrition and Your Health: Dietary Guidelines for Americans." Free.
- "Thrifty Meals for Two." Aprox. $2.50.
- "Some Facts and Myths About Vitamins." Free.

Consumer Reports

The magazine *Consumer Reports* has numerous articles, reprints, and books on health topics. There is an excellent article, "Medicare-Supplemental Insurance," in the June 1984 issue (p. 347). Reprints cost $1.00. For reprints, write:

Reprints
Consumer Reports
P.O. Box 1949
Marion, OH 43305

Some other *Consumer Reports* reprints of interest include the following:

- "Diet and Heart Disease"
- "Caffeine: What It Does; How to Consume Less"
- "Arthritis: Treatment and Mistreatment"
- "Too Much Sugar?"

For *Consumer Reports* books, write to:

Consumer Reports Books
Box C-719
Brooklyn, NY 11205

The following are some books of interest from *Consumer Reports*:

- *Drug Information for the Consumer*. By authority of the United States Pharmacopeial Convention, Inc. 1978. 1,224 pages, paperbound. Approx. $25.00.
- *Understanding Arthritis*. By the Arthritis Foundation. 304 pages. Paper. Approx. $11.00
- *Physical Fitness for Practically Everybody*. 1983. 336 pages. Paper. Approx. $12.95.
- *The Columbia University Complete Home Medical Guide*. 928 pages. 1985. Paper. Approx. $25.00.
- *Straight-talk, No-nonsense Guide to Heart Care*. Developed by the American Medical Association. 1984. 210 pages. Paper. $11.00.
- *Vitamins and Minerals: Help or Harm?* Revised, 1985. 272 pages. Approx. $13.00.
- *The Home Health Care Solution*. 1985. 448 pages. Paper. Approx. $12.00.
- *Living with Dying*. 400 pages. 1985. Paper. Approx. $13.00.

To subscribe to *Consumer Reports* magazine, write:

Consumer Reports
P.O. Box 2480
Boulder, CO 80322

The American Association of Retired Persons (AARP)

You do not have to be a member of AARP to take advantage of their free booklets or to purchase many of their products. However, membership is only $5.00 per year, and members enjoy discounts.

To order *multiple copies* of booklets or for general information, write:

American Association of Retired Persons
1909 K Street, N.W.
Washington, DC 20049

For *single copies* of booklets, write:

American Association of Retired Persons
Box 2400
Long Beach, CA 90801

The following booklets are available free of charge from AARP:

- "Housing Options for Older Americans," Order No. D12063.
- "A Handbook About Care in the Home," Order No. D955.
- "Eating for Your Good Health," Order No. D12164.
- "Information on Medicare and Health Insurance," Order No. C38.
- "Miles Away and Still Caring: A Guide for Long-Distance Caregivers," Order No. D12748. This AARP booklet lists addresses and phone numbers of all state units on aging, which are required by law to offer information and referral services free of charge. The State Units on Aging are able to refer you to your local Area Agency on Aging, which in turn can give you information about local resources in your particular community.

To order any AARP book, write:

AARP Books,
c/o Scott, Foresman and Company
1865 Miner St.
Des Plaines, IL 60016

You must add $1.75 per total order (*not* per book) to cover shipping and handling. To order a catalogue of AARP books, write:

AARP Books
1900 East Lake Avenue
Glenview, IL 60025

If buying at your local bookstore (by special order), it may help to specify that the distributor is Farrar, Straus and Giroux.

The following is a selected list of particularly valuable AARP books for senior citizens:

- *The Gadget Book: Ingenious Devices for Easier Living*, edited by Dennis R. La Buda for the American Society on Aging. 1985. Order No. 673-24819-4. $10.95. (Reviewed later in this chapter on page 294.)
- *Caregiving: Helping an Aging Loved One*, by Jo Horne. Order No. 673-24822-4. $13.95.
- *Cataracts: The Complete Guide—from Diagnosis to Recovery—for Patients and Families*, by Julius Shulman, M.D. Order No. 673-2448244-0. $7.95.
- *Fitness for Life: Exercises for People Over 50*, by Theodore Berland. Order No. 673-24823-7. $12.95.
- *National Continuing Care Directory: Retirement Communities with Prepaid Medical Plans*, edited by Ann Trueblood Raper. Order No. 673-24813-5. $13.95.
- *The Over Easy Foot Care Book*, by Timothy P. Shea, D.P.M., and Joan K. Smith. Order No. 673-24807-0. $6.95.
- *Policy Wise: The Practical Guide to Insurance Decisions for Older Consumers*, by Nancy H. Chasen. Order No. 673-24806-2.
- *Survival Handbook for Widows (and for Relatives and Friends Who Want to Understand)*, by Ruth J. Loewinsohn. Order No. 673-248820-8. $5.95.

Metropolitan Life Insurance Company

The following free pamphlets are available from the Metropolitan Life Insurance Company

- "Alcohol and Health"
- "Exercise"
- "Healthy Aging"
- "Hearing Impairments"
- "How You Can Control Your Weight"
- "Immunizations—When and Why"
- "Personal Health Record"
- "Vision Care"

Order from:

> Metropolitan Life Insurance Company
> Health and Safety Education Division
> One Madison Avenue
> New York, NY 10010

Newsletters

Various organizations publish a number of newsletters on health subjects of interest to senior citizens. These are typically published on a quarterly basis. Other, freestanding newsletters are typically published monthly.

The Arthritis Foundation publishes a bi-monthly magazine, *Arthritis Today*. To subscribe, write:

> The Arthritis Foundation
> National Office
> 1314 Spring Street, N.W.
> Atlanta, GA 30309

The American Society on Aging publishes a quarterly journal, *Generations*, which focuses on topics of interest to senior citizens. It is available for $20.00 per year by writing to:

> Generations
> 833 Market Street, Suite 516
> San Francisco, CA 94103

Back issues of *Generations* are available for $2.00 to $7.00 each.

The National Support Center for Families of the Aging (listed earlier in this chapter) has a quarterly newsletter called *Change* ($10.00 per year), which provides ideas, updates, and information on caregiving.

The Tufts University School of Medicine publishes *The Tufts University Diet and Nutrition Letter*. To subscribe, write:

> Tufts University Diet and Nutrition Letter
> Subscription Department
> P.O. Box 10948
> Des Moines, IA 50950

A consumer group called The Public Citizen Health Research Group publishes the monthly *Health Letter*, available for $18.00 per year. To subscribe, write:

> Health Letter
> P.O. Box 19404
> Washington, DC 20077-6488

Another consumer group publishes *The Nutrition Action Newsletter*. Price is $19.95 per year. To subscribe, write:

Center for Science in the Public Interest
P.O. Box 33759
Washington, DC 20077-5932

The University of California, Berkeley, publishes an excellent newsletter, *The Wellness Letter*. A subscription is $20.00 per year. Write:

University of California, Berkeley Wellness Letter
Subscription Dept.
P.O. Box 10935
Des Moines, IA 50340

The *Harvard Medical School Health Letter* costs $16.00 per year. To subscribe, write:

Harvard Medical School Health Letter
Subscription Services
P.O. Box 10944
Des Moines, IA 50340

The *Mayo Clinic Health Letter* costs $24.00 per year. To subscribe, write:

Mayo Clinic Health Letter
Mayo Medical Resources
Rochester, MN 55905

A San Francisco Bay Area family physician turned radio and television personality—Dr. Dean Edell—now publishes the *Edell Health Letter* ($24.00 a year). To subscribe, write The Edell Health Letter, P.O. Box 50162, Boulder, CO 80321-0162. It keeps its readers up to date on current health findings garnered from more than 150 medical journals. The purpose is to present the same studies and research that your doctor reads, but in plain, down-to-earth language. It also contains information that does not appear in other health magazines.

Books

In addition to those books already listed under other headings, here are some titles of particular interest to senior citizens and their caregivers:

- *Self-Care and Self-Help Groups for the Elderly: A Directory*, available from:

  National Institute on Aging/SCSH
  2209 Distribution Circle
  Silver Spring, MD 20910
  (301) 495-3455

- *The Age Care Sourcebook: A Resource Guide for the Aging and Their Families*, by Jean Crichton (Fireside Books/Simon & Schuster, 1987). $9.95.
- *The Pill Book: The Illustrated Guide to the Most Prescribed Drugs in the United States*, by Harold M. Silverman and Gilbert I. Simon. (Bantam Books, 1986). $12.95.
- *The Essential Guide to Non-Prescription Drugs*, by David R. Zimmerman (Harper & Row, 1983). $10.95.
- *The Complete Home Medical Guide*, by The Columbia University College of Physicians and Surgeons. (Crown Books, 1985). Hardcover, $39.95.
- *American Heart Association Heartbook* (E.P. Dutton, 1980) $25.00.
- *American Cancer Society Cancer Book* (Doubleday, 1986) $22.50.
- *Handbook of Nutrition, Health and Aging*, by Donald M. Watkin. (Park Ridge, N.J.: Noyes Publications, 1983).
- *Handbook for the Elderly and Handicapped*, by Jean Sargent. (Ames: Iowa State University Press, 1981).
- *The 36-Hour Day: A Family Guide to Caring for Persons with Alzheimer's Disease, Related Dementing Illnesses, and Memory Loss in Later Life*, by Nancy Mace and Peter V. Rabins, M.D. (N.Y.: Warner Books, 1981).
- *How to Select a Nursing Home*, U.S. Dept. of Health and Human Services. (Baltimore, Md: Health Care Financing Administration, 1980).
- *A Consumer Guide to Hospice Care*, by Barbara Coleman. (Washington, D.C.: National Consumers League, 1985).
- *Family Caregiving and Dependent Elderly*, by Dianne Springer and Timothy Brubaker. (Beverly Hills, Calif.: Sage Publications, 1984).

Health Libraries

The following institutions either are libraries or have libraries which specialize in consumer health information:

American Academy of Family
  Physicians
8880 Ward Parkway
Kansas City, MO 64114-0723

Center for Medical Consumers
237 Thompson St.
New York, NY 10012

Consumer Health Information
  Center
680 East 600 South
Salt Lake City, UT 84102

Community Health Information
  Network (CHIN)
330 Mt. Auburn St.
Cambridge, MA 62238

Consumer Health Information
  Project and Services (CHIPS)
Carson Public Library
151 E. Carson St.
Carson, CA 90745

Harbor-UCLA Medical Center
A.F. Parlow Library, Box 18
1000 W. Carson
Torrance, CA 90509

Health Education Center
200 Ross St.
Pittsburgh, PA 15219

Health Library
Kaiser-Permanente Medical
  Center
280 W. MacArthur Blvd., 12th
  Floor
Oakland, CA 94611

Planetree Health Resource Center
2040 Webster St.
San Francisco, CA 94115

Sisters of St. Mary National Family
  Practice Research and
  Development Center
2900 Baltimore
Kansas City, MO 64108

Gadgets

An astounding number of "gadgets" can make life easier for senior citizens. A most useful listing is provided in the AARP book, *The Gadget Book: Ingenious Devices for Easier Living* (ordering details listed on page 289). The book lists hundreds of gadgets, with an appendix cross-referencing them according to 32 "Activities of Daily Living." Also listed are 296 manufacturers and distributors. Some especially useful gadgets include the following:

- High-sided dish or bowl (to prevent spilling)
- Rocker knife (to aid cutting food with only one hand)
- Shoe aid (plastic insert slips on back of shoe to prevent bending while slipping foot in)
- Elevated toilet seat
- Bathtub safety treads
- Shower chair or stool
- Grab bar for shower, bathtub, or toilet

- Catapult chair (lifts the person up to a standing from the sitting position)
- Phosphorescent tape (to mark switches, doorknobs, etc.)
- Sound-activated light switch (turns on with a clap of the hands)
- Burn-proof kettle (automatically shuts off when empty)
- Reacher tongs (for grabbing cans or other objects from high shelves)
- Auxiliary telephone dialer with large buttons
- Telephone adapter for the hearing impaired (amplifier)
- Emergency alert system/call-for-help telephone (pendant worn around neck can automatically dial one or more predetermined phone numbers with prerecorded message to send for help)
- Attachments for walker (in which to carry objects)
- Pill organizer (box with four compartments for each day, and seven rows of compartments for each day of the week)
- Large-print books
- Hand-held magnifying glass

Other catalogues of "gadgets" can be obtained by writing to:

Independent Living Aids, Inc.
27 East Mall
Plainview, NY 11803
(516) 752-8080

Vis-Aids, Inc.
102-09 Jamaica Avenue
P.O. Box 26
Richmond Hill, NY 11418
(718) 847-4734 or 441-2550

Facile Fashions (clothing with velcro fastenings instead of buttons)
Box 10510
Rochester, NY 14610 (catalogue $1.00)

A "Personal Home Care Catalogue" of home care products available by mail is produced by the AARP Pharmacy Service. The catalogue can be obtained by writing to the AARP's Washington, D.C. address (listed on page 266) or to:

AARP Home Care Center
3557 Lafayette Road
Indianapolis, IN 46222

Another catalogue of health products for the disabled elderly is available from:

CarePoint
Catalogue Division
50 Tiburon Street
San Rafael, CA 94901
1-800-334-8999 weekdays 10 A.M. to 4 P.M.

Some typical products listed are:

- Folding cane
- Ultrasonic humidifier
- Trigger action reacher (mechanical gripper which also has magnet for small metal objects)
- Folding cane

Toll-Free Numbers and Hotlines

One can call a number of toll-free numbers for health and other information of interest to senior citizens. Some of these numbers are listed here.

To order any book by mail 24 hours a day (have your credit card ready) call:

1-800-255-2665
1-800-C[A]LL-BOOK
[in Connecticut or worldwide, call (203)966-5470]
(Book Call)

1-800-635-0045 (Books of All Publishers)
1-800-248-8886 (Discount Books by Phone)

The Cancer Information Service number (sponsored by the National Cancer Institute) is:

1-800-4-CANCER
Alaska 1-800-638-6070
Washington, D.C. and suburbs 635-5700
Oahu 524-1234 (call collect from neighboring islands)

For general information on cancer and cancer services, call:

1-800-525-3777
(AMC Cancer Research Center, Denver)

For breast self-examination information, call:

800-MAM-CARE

For information regarding *early detection of bowel cancer* call:

1-800-ED-HELPS

For materials on alcoholism aimed at families, call:

1-800-356-9996
(Al-Anon Family Group Headquarters)

For printed information on alcoholism and referral to local affiliates, call:

1-800-NCA-CALL
(National Council on Alcoholism)

For free information and literature about diabetes, call:

1-800-232-3472
(American Diabetes Assn.)
(8:30 A.M. to 5 P.M. eastern time)

For information on rehabilitation, including assistive devices, call:

1-800-34-NARIC
(National Rehabilitation Center)
(9 A.M. to 5 P.M. eastern time)

For information on hearing problems and referral to local numbers for a 2-minute hearing test (also answers questions on broken hearing aids, and makes referrals to local ear/nose/throat specialists), call:

1-800-222-EARS
1-800-345-EARS in PA
(Dial a Hearing Test)
(9 A.M. to 6 P.M. eastern time)

For information on heart disease and pacemakers, call:

1-800-241-6993
(404) 523-0826 in Georgia
(Heartlife)
(9 A.M. to 4 P.M. eastern time)

For information on chronic bronchitis and emphysema, call:

1-800-222-5864
(303) 355-LUNG in Denver
(Lung Line, National Asthma Center)
(8 A.M. to 5 P.M. mountain time)

For information on free eye exams for senior citizens who are financially disadvantaged and have not seen an ophthalmologist for at least three years, call:

1-800-222-EYES
(National Eye Care Project Helpline)
(5 A.M. to 5 P.M. Pacific time)

For questions about incontinence and its management, provided by Procter & Gamble, call:

1-800-4-ATTENDS

The Simon Foundation, a nonprofit education and informational organization for persons who suffer from incontinence, also has a toll-free hotline for questions about incontinence:

1-800-23-SIMON

For information on publications about Alzheimer's disease, call:

1-800-621-0379
[Illinois residents, call (800) 572-6037]

For general information about life and health insurance, the American Council of Life Insurance and the Health Insurance Association of America sponsors a toll-free number:

1-800-432-8000
[In the Washington, D.C. area (202) 862-4054]

Information about calcium and the prevention of osteoporosis is available from the Dallas Osteoporosis Center; call:

1-800-722-BONE

The *Silver Pages Directory* lists businesses and services that cater to persons age 60 and older. It also lists businesses that offer discounts or free services to older persons. It is free to those who live in the area it covers. To order, call:

1-800-252-6050

Chapter 32

A CHECKLIST

As suggested in the introduction to this handbook, there are two distinct aspects to the practice of modern medicine: crisis care and preventive medicine. In a very real sense, they tend to be mutually exclusive: those who plan ahead are far less likely to encounter medical crises, while those whose health suffers the most tend to be persons who never bothered to do much in the way of preventive care. While no one can *entirely* avoid medical crises—indeed, everyone must someday face that *ultimate* health crisis—death—those who *do* plan ahead by choosing wise health habits early in life will be much less likely to find frequent "surprises" cropping up in their later years. It is the goal of this book to assist those who would like to *avoid* such "surprises" as much as possible. By learning which crises are most likely to strike after 65, one can have a better perspective from which to begin a sensible program of diet, exercise, and good health maintenance habits. Such a program cannot guarantee a long and healthy life, but it will at least give you a "fighting chance" to achieve that goal.

In this handbook, we have presented a wide array of periodic examinations one may wish to consider. In addition, we have suggested certain documents to obtain for emergency or routine use. In this chapter, we list them all together by way of reminder. We emphasize the most important examinations with **boldface** type. In addition, those examinations which generally should be done at least annually from age 50 to 70 have their checkboxes enhanced with **bold lines.** Page references are given for ease of reviewing the reasoning behind the exams and the specifics of carrying them out.

This checklist can be used by patients and doctors alike as a way of keeping track of the baffling array of health maintenance examinations which are germane to adults of various ages. It is recommended that one review this checklist annually. Many people find themselves most amenable to considering these recommendations around the time of the New Year, when resolutions are often made to do better in the future.

Since only a small percentage of people bother with even the least controversial exams—such as mammograms or stool testing for blood—there is little danger of placing *too much emphasis* on this sort of health maintenance checklist. Furthermore, the temporary demise of the annual pap smear—because of a recent change in recommendations by the American Cancer Society, which was reversed only a few months later—has been interpreted by many women as a reason not to see their doctor for *other* periodic examinations between times. Aside from the fact that the annual Pap smear *has* been reinstated, such behavior—as this checklist outlines—is not consistent with fastidious health maintenance.

Home Examinations
- **Monthly breast self-exam** (women) (pages 24–25)   ☐
- Periodic self-examination of other areas (pages 32–33)
  —thyroid   ☐
  —testicles (men)   ☐
  —lymph nodes   ☐
  —oral region   ☐
  —skin   ☐
- **Self-testing of stool for occult blood:** all men and women   ☐
  should have three tests of stool for microscopic blood
  every two years from age 40 to 50, and annually after that
  (pages 28–31).

Medical History
- **Comprehensive data base:** done initially (pages 232–234,   ☐
  307–313)
- **Periodic update: the history** should be updated every   ☐
  five years from age 20 to 60, every 2½ years from age 61
  to 75, and annually after age 75 (page 234).

Physical Exam by Primary Doctor
- **Comprehensive examination:** done initially. ☐
- **Periodic update:** a **physical examination,** including meas- ☐
  urement of **weight** and **blood pressure,** should be done
  every five years from age 20 to 60, every 2½ years from
  age 61 to 75, and annually after age 75 (page 234).
  - —**additional blood pressure readings:** should be taken at ☐
    2½-year intervals between the above exams from age
    20 to 60 (page 234).
  - —**rectal exam:** should be done beginning at age 40 (page ☐
    31).
  - —**breast exam** (women): a doctor's examination of the ☐
    breasts should be performed every two years until age
    50, and then once a year after that (page 24).
  - —**pelvic exam** (women): should be done annually on all ☐
    women who have every been sexually active or who
    have reached the age of 18 (pages 28, 32).
  - —**Pap smear** (women): should be done annually on all ☐
    women who have ever been sexually active or who have
    reached the age of 18. After three consecutive satisfac-
    tory normal annual examinations, the Pap test may be
    performed less frequently, at the physician's discre-
    tion. (pages 27–28)
  - —**sigmoidoscopy** (**often done by a gastroenterologist**): ☐
    recommended every three to five years after two an-
    nual negatives, starting at age 50 (page 31).

Physical Exams by Specialists
- Complete eye exam: every two to four years is a reason- ☐
  able schedule for persons over 40 without specific eye
  problems (page 237).
- Glaucoma screening by an ophthalmologist: should begin ☐
  at age 40 and continue at least every two years thereafter,
  and more frequently if measurements are borderline
  normal or if there is a positive family history of glaucoma
  (page 236).
- Hearing exam: should be conducted in the case of hearing ☐
  difficulty once obvious correctable causes—especially
  wax plugs—have been ruled out (pages 130–132).

- Dental exam: semi-annual checkups are important at all ☐ ages while any teeth remain; annual checkups are recommended for those without teeth. (page 140)

Laboratory and X-ray Tests
- **Testing of stool for occult blood:** all men and women ☐ should have three tests of stool for microscopic blood every two years from age 40 to 50, and annually after that. Even if a doctor does one testing of stool for occult blood with the rectal exam at the time of an annual physical, at least two additional tests should be performed by the patient beyond this. (pages 30–31)
- **Chest x-ray:** a baseline chest x-ray should be done at age ☐ 40 (page 234).
- **Mammogram:** all women should have a baseline mam- ☐ mogram between age 35 to 39, and then periodic mammograms every year or two from age 40 to 50, and annually after age 50 (pages 24–27).
- **EKG:** a baseline EKG should be done at ages 20, 40, and ☐ 60 (page 234).
- Blood tests
  —**complete blood count** (page 235)   ☐
  —**cholesterol level:** cholesterol levels optional after age ☐ 60, depending on the previous results. Should be done every five years from age 20 to 60. (page 234)
  —**triglycerides level:** (fasting) triglyceride levels optional ☐ after age 60, depending on the previous results. Should be done every five years from age 20 to 60. (page 234)
  —**fasting blood sugar:** optional after age 75, depending ☐ on previous results. Should be done every five years from age 20 to 60, and every 2½ years from age 61 to 75. (page 234)
  —**chemistry panel** (page 235)   ☐
  —**thyroid functions tests** (page 235)   ☐
  —**syphilis test:** should be done once, as part of the data ☐ base (page 235).
- Urine analysis (page 235).   ☐

Special Evaluations
- **Osteoporosis Evaluation at (optimally) or After Onset of** ☐ **Menopause** (women) (pages 82–83)

- **Evaluation for Regular Use of Aspirin to Prevent Heart Attacks.** All men and those women with "risk factors" (smoking, high blood pressure, high cholesterol, positive family history of heart attacks, diabetes, etc.) might well be advised to take one regular strength aspirin (325 mg) every other day between age 35 and 70. (pages 14–15) ☐

Immunizations (pages 239–241)
- **Tetanus booster:** should be continued every ten years as an adult if one has had the primary series in childhood. ☐
- **Diphtheria booster:** should be continued every ten years as an adult if one has had the primary series in childhood ☐
- **Flu vaccination:** recommended for all adults over 65. The best time is from September through December. ☐
- **Pneumococcal vaccination:** recommended *once* for all adults over 65. ☐

Personal Medical Documentation
- **Wallet card with basic medical information** (page 247) ☐
- **Wallet card with baseline EKG** (page 248) ☐
- **Wallet card with living will and/or addendum *or* list of agent and alternatives for durable power of attorney** (pages 248–254, 257–258) ☐
- **Copy of living will and/or addendum *or* list of agent and alternatives for durable power of attorney *on file with primary care doctor*** (pages 248, 254, 257–58) ☐
- **Family health record** (to bring to initial comprehensive history-taking encounter and to all subsequent comprehensive periodic exams for updating any interval changes) (page 249). ☐
- Personal medication record (to bring to all doctor visits) (page 249). ☐

Counseling
Seatbelt Use Awareness (page 235) ☐
Home Safety Check (pages 77, 235) ☐
Health Counseling About Cancer Prevention and Detection. Every three years, starting at age 20, and annually from age 40 on (page 32). ☐

APPENDICES

Appendix A

PATIENT'S HEALTH SURVEY QUESTIONNAIRE

The following questions pertain to information that doctors need most from their patients. You might wish—if your doctor agrees— to bring in the completed questionnaire at the time of a comprehensive exam, as it can greatly facilitate the history-taking process.

YES NO

1. Are you allergic to any medicines that you know of? ___ ___

2. Have any other medicines ever caused you to have a bad reaction? ___ ___

3. Have you ever had your tonsils out? ___ ___

4. (For women only) Have you had your uterus removed (a hysterectomy)? ___ ___

5. (For women only) Have you ever had your bladder "lifted"? ___ ___

6. (For women only) Have you ever had your tubes tied (to become sterile)? ___ ___

7. Have you ever had your gallbladder out? ___ ___

8. Have you ever had your appendix removed? ___ ___

9. Have you ever had a hernia operation? ___ ___

10. Have you ever had cataract surgery? ___ ___

11. Have you ever had any other operation on your eyes? ___ ___

12. Have you ever had any skin lesions removed? ___ ___

13. Have you ever had any other operations or surgical procedures? ___ ___

14. Have you ever suffered a serious blow to your head?

YES NO

15. Have you ever broken any bones, such as ribs, shoulders, arms, wrists, hands, legs, ankles, or feet? ___ ___

16. Have you ever injured yourself in any other way, including "whiplash" injury to your neck, or sprained your shoulder, back, or ankle? ___ ___

17. Have you ever had the mumps? ___ ___

18. Have you ever had the "regular" measles? ___ ___

19. Have you ever had the "German" measles? ___ ___

20. Have you ever had chicken pox? ___ ___

21. Did you have any other childhood diseases? ___ ___

22. Did you *miss* any of the usual childhood "shots" and immunizations for diphtheria, tetanus, whooping cough, mumps, measles, and polio? ___ ___

23. Did you ever have any X-ray treatment to your face, neck, or chest, even in childhood? ___ ___

24. Have you had a tetanus shot within the past 10 years? ___ ___

25. Have you had a diphtheria shot within the past 10 years? (If it were given, generally it would be combined with a tetanus booster.) ___ ___

307

YES NO

26. Have you ever had a flu shot? ___ ___

27. Have you ever had a vaccination against pneumonia? ___ ___

28. Have you ever had a TB skin test? ___ ___

29. Have you ever been told that you had rheumatic fever? ___ ___

30. Have you ever been told that you had a heart murmur? ___ ___

31. Have you ever had high blood pressure? ___ ___

32. Have you ever had pneumonia? ___ ___

33. Have you ever had a heart attack? ___ ___

34. Have you ever had gonorrhea? ___ ___

35. Have you ever had syphilis ("bad blood")? ___ ___

36. (For women only) Have you ever had infection in your tubes? ___ ___

37. Have you ever had, or been told you had, genital herpes? ___ ___

38. Have you ever had, or been told you had, venereal warts? ___ ___

39. Have you ever had any other sexually transmitted disease? ___ ___

40. Have you ever had hepatitis? ___ ___

41. Have you ever had a transfusion? ___ ___

42. (For women only) Have you ever had any children? ___ ___

43. (For women only) Have you ever had a miscarriage or an abortion? ___ ___

44. (For women only) If you have had any children, did you ever breast feed any of them? ___ ___

45. Have you had a blood or urine test in the last few years? ___ ___

46. Have you had a complete physical in the last few years? ___ ___

47. (For women only) Have you had a Pap smear in the last three years? ___ ___

48. (For women only) Have you ever had an abnormal Pap smear? ___ ___

49. Has a doctor ever looked inside your rectum with a long lighted tube? ___ ___

50. Have you ever had a biopsy? ___ ___

51. Have you ever had a chest X-ray? ___ ___

52. Have you ever had an EKG? ___ ___

53. (For women only) Do you *fail* to examine your breasts carefully each month? ___ ___

54. (For women only) Have you had a mammogram (X-ray of the breasts) in the last 12 months? ___ ___

YES NO

55. (For women only) Have you *ever* had a mammogram? ___ ___

56. Have you ever had an X-ray of your large intestine (barium enema)? ___ ___

57. Have you ever had an X-ray of your stomach (upper GI series)? ___ ___

58. Have you ever had an X-ray of your gallbladder? ___ ___

59. Have you ever had an X-ray of your kidneys? ___ ___

60. Have you ever had any other photographic medical studies, such as a "CAT scan" or Ultrasound? ___ ___

61. Have you ever had any radiation *treatments*? ___ ___

62. Have you ever had thyroid cancer? ___ ___

63. Have you ever had cancer of the larynx (voice box)? ___ ___

64. Have you ever had cancer anywhere in the mouth or throat? ___ ___

65. Have you ever had emphysema? ___ ___

66. Have you ever had lung cancer? ___ ___

67. Have you ever had cancer of the kidney? ___ ___

68. Have you ever had cancer of the bladder (not the gallbladder)? ___ ___

69. Have you ever had polyps in the stomach (not the large intestine)? ___ ___

70. Have you ever been told that you had *pernicious anemia*? ___ ___

71. Have you ever had stomach cancer? ___ ___

72. Have you ever had polyps in the large intestine or the bowels or the rectum? ___ ___

73. Have you ever had a condition called *ulcerative colitis*? ___ ___

74. Have you ever had cancer of the large intestine? ___ ___

75. Have you ever had skin cancer? ___ ___

76. (For women only) Have you ever had sexual intercourse? ___ ___

77. (For women only) Did your mother ever use the female hormone DES (diethylstilbestrol) when she was pregnant with you? ___ ___

78. (For women only) Have you ever had cancer of the cervix? ___ ___

79. (For women only) Have you ever had cancer of the uterus? ___ ___

80. (For women only) Have you ever had cancer of the vagina? ___ ___

81. (For women only) Have you ever had breast cancer? ___ ___

YES NO

82. Have you ever been hospitalized? ___ ___
83. Have you ever been married? ___ ___
84. Do you live alone? ___ ___
85. Do you prepare your own meals? ___ ___
86. Do you eat fried foods regularly? ___ ___
87. Do you eat more than one egg per week? ___ ___
88. Do you eat pork regularly? ___ ___
89. Do you add a lot of salt to your food? ___ ___
90. Do you eat bran-containing cereal regularly? ___ ___
91. Do you now smoke? ___ ___
92. Have you ever smoked? ___ ___
93. Do you now drink alcohol in any form? ___ ___
94. Have you ever in the past used alcohol in any form? ___ ___
95. Is it difficult for you to go shopping for food? ___ ___
96. Is it difficult for you to afford the kinds of foods you think you should eat? ___ ___
97. Do you think you need help handling your financial affairs? ___ ___
98. Do you have any relatives who take an interest in your welfare? ___ ___
99. Do you have any friends who would take an interest in your welfare? ___ ___
100. Do you have Medicare? ___ ___
101. Would you wish to have **cardiopulmonary resuscitation** (doctors trying to re-start your heart by pumping on your breastbone and breathing into your mouth) if your heart should stop during a terminal condition (one where you were not expected to live six months) and you could not communicate your wishes? ___ ___
102. Would you wish to be **intubated** (have a breathing tube passed into your lungs) to improve your breathing if you should develop a terminal condition and could not communicate your wishes? ___ ___
103. Would you wish to be **fed through a tube** if you should develop a terminal condition where you could no longer eat sufficiently in the normal way and could not communicate your wishes? ___ ___
104. Would you wish to be given **intravenous fluids** if you should develop a terminal condition and could not communicate your wishes? ___ ___
105. Would you wish to be given **intravenous or intramuscular antibiotics** to

YES NO

prolong your life if you should develop a terminal condition and could not communicate your wishes? ___ ___
106. Would you wish to be **hospitalized** to prolong your life if you should develop a terminal condition and could not communicate your wishes? ___ ___
107. Would you wish to have **cardiopulmonary resuscitation** if you should become severely demented and could not communicate your wishes? ___ ___
108. Would you wish to be **intubated** (have a breathing tube passed into your lungs) to improve your breathing if you should become severely demented and could not communicate your wishes? ___ ___
109. Would you wish to be **fed through a tube** if you should become severely demented and could no longer eat sufficiently in the normal way and could not communicate your wishes? ___ ___
110. Would you wish to be given **intravenous fluids** if you should become severely demented and could not communicate your wishes? ___ ___
111. Would you wish to be given **intravenous or intramuscular antibiotics** if you should become severely demented and could not communicate your wishes? ___ ___
112. Would you wish to be **hospitalized** to prolong your life if you should become severely demented and could not communicate your wishes? ___ ___
113. Do you take Anacin, Bufferin, or aspirin regularly? ___ ___
114. Do you sometimes take antacids such as Maalox, Tums, or Rolaids? ___ ___
115. Do you sometimes take a pill for upset stomach? ___ ___
116. Do you sometimes take pain pills, including aspirin, Anacin, Bufferin, Tylenol, Advil, Nuprin, or Medipren? ___ ___
117. Do you sometimes take sleeping pills? ___ ___
118. Do you ever take "allergy" pills? ___ ___
119. Do you ever take "sinus" pills? ___ ___
120. Do you ever take asthma pills? ___ ___
121. Have you ever used a hand-held breathing device for asthma? ___ ___
122. Have you ever taken pills for high blood pressure? ___ ___
123. Have you ever taken potassium pills or liquid? ___ ___

YES NO   YES NO

124. Do you eat bananas or drink orange juice or eat any other potassium-rich foods on the advice of a doctor?   — —

125. Do you take a heart pill?   — —

126. Have you ever taken water pills?   — —

127. Have you ever taken thyroid pills?   — —

128. Have you ever taken a pill under the tongue for chest pain?   — —

129. Have you ever used a medicated strip of salve placed on your skin to relieve chest pain?   — —

130. Have you ever used any other kind of medicated strip of salve placed on your skin at regular intervals?   — —

131. Have you ever taken any kind of pills to improve your circulation?   — —

132. Have you ever taken pills for diabetes?   — —

133. Have you ever taken insulin?   — —

134. Have you ever taken any pills for convulsions or seizures?   — —

135. (For women only) Have you ever taken birth control pills?   — —

136. (For women only) Have you ever had female hormone therapy for treatment of menopausal symptoms?   — —

137. (For women only) Have you ever taken female hormone pills to prevent osteoporosis?   — —

138. Have you ever taken nerve pills?   — —

139. Have you ever taken sleeping pills?   — —

140. Have you ever taken diet pills?   — —

141. (For women only) Have you ever used a device inside the uterus for birth control?   — —

142. Do you sometimes use a salve or cream on your skin, or over your joints?   — —

143. (For women only) Have you had to use a cream or suppository for your genital area in the past year or two?   — —

144. Have you had to use a salve or suppository for your rectum in the past year or two?   — —

145. Do you sometimes take vitamins?   — —

146. Do you sometimes take iron pills or vitamin pills that contain iron?   — —

147. Do you regularly take calcium pills?   — —

148. Do you use laxatives sometimes?   — —

149. Do you sometimes give yourself enemas?   — —

150. Do you sometimes take medicine to soften your bowel movements?   — —

151. Do you use any eye or ear drops on a daily basis?   — —

152. Do you take certain eye or ear drops from time to time, as needed, for particular problems?   — —

153. Is there any diabetes in your family?   — —

154. Has anyone in your family had an amputation?   — —

155. Is there high blood pressure in your family?   — —

156. Has anyone in your family had a heart attack?   — —

157. Has anyone in your family been born with a heart problem?   — —

158. Has anyone in your family had a heart murmur?   — —

159. Has anyone in your family ever used pills under the tongue for chest pain?   — —

160. Has anyone in your family ever had a stroke?   — —

161. (For women only) Have any of your female blood relatives had breast cancer?   — —

162. Have any of your blood relatives had stomach cancer?   — —

163. Have any of your blood relatives ever had colon or bowel polyps?   — —

164. Have any of your blood relatives ever had cancer of the colon or the large intestine?   — —

165. (For women only) Have any of your female blood relatives had uterine or cervical cancer (cancer of the womb)?   — —

166. Is there any other history of cancer in your family?   — —

167. Has anyone in your family ever had problems with the thyroid gland?   — —

168. Has anyone in your family ever had kidney stones?   — —

169. Has anyone in your family ever had gallstones?   — —

170. Has anyone in your family ever had TB?   — —

171. Has anyone in your family ever had glaucoma?   — —

172. Has anyone in your family ever had asthma, hay fever, allergies, or a reaction to penicillin?   — —

173. Has anyone in your family ever had any other illnesses not mentioned above?   — —

174. Has anyone in your family committed suicide?   — —

YES NO YES NO

175. Do you have difficulty walking about and climbing stairs without using a cane or other assistive device? ___ ___

176. Do you often suffer from the fear that you may fall down? ___ ___

177. Have you fallen down in the past year? ___ ___

178. Have you had problems with dizziness lately? ___ ___

179. Do you feel tired and don't know why? ___ ___

180. Do you sometimes get dizzy for a moment when you first stand up?

181. Have you suffered unexplained weight loss of more than 10 lb in the past six months? ___ ___

182. Has your appetite diminished recently? ___ ___

183. Have you noticed a lump in your breasts or elsewhere? ___ ___

184. Has there been any bleeding or change in size or in color of any moles during the past six months? ___ ___

185. Has there been any bleeding or change in the size of a wart during the past six months? ___ ___

186. Do you now suffer from a sore that has been present for at least one month? ___ ___

187. Have you noticed any skin changes in an area where you had X-ray treatment at one time? ___ ___

188. Is there a bad scar somewhere on your body from a burn which happened at least a year ago? ___ ___

189. Do you have any moles on the soles of your feet or your palms, or someplace where irritation by clothing or jewelry may occur? ___ ___

190. Do you have very fair skin and/or sunburn easily? ___ ___

191. Have you noticed a rash anywhere lately? ___ ___

192. Have you had itching "all over" lately? ___ ___

193. Have you had itching in your rectum or around your genital area lately? ___ ___

194. Do you get headaches frequently? ___ ___

195. Do you tend to get "sinus" pains around your eyes, forehead, or face from time to time? ___ ___

196. Do you wear glasses? ___ ___

197. Do you wear contact lenses? ___ ___

198. Do your eyes itch often? ___ ___

199. Do your eyes water often? ___ ___

200. Has your eyesight gotten poor? ___ ___

201. Is your hearing not what it should be? ___ ___

202. Have you ever had your hearing tested? ___ ___

203. Are your ears often stuffy? ___ ___

204. Do your ears itch often? ___ ___

205. Is there a discharge from either of your ears? ___ ___

206. Do you get a ringing or noise in your ears sometimes? ___ ___

207. Do you get a runny or stuffy nose often? ___ ___

208. Do you get nosebleeds often? ___ ___

209. Are you aware of any cavities in your teeth at this time? ___ ___

210. Do you have irritation of your tongue, cheek, or gums caused by dentures or a tooth? ___ ___

211. Have you suffered from pain or tenderness in your mouth for at least a month? ___ ___

212. Have you noticed a sore or a white spot inside your mouth, on your tongue, or on your lips that has lasted more than a month? ___ ___

213. Have you noticed any hoarseness or voice changes which have lasted more than a month? ___ ___

214. Have you suffered from a steady pressure or tightness in the front of the lower part of your neck that has lasted more than a month? ___ ___

215. Have you been coughing daily for more than a month? ___ ___

216. Have you coughed up any blood in the past month? ___ ___

217. Do you often get chest congestion, either at night or during the day? ___ ___

218. Do you sometimes get wheezing in your chest? ___ ___

219. Have you been coughing up anything lately? ___ ___

220. Have you had any other problems with your breathing? ___ ___

221. (For women only) Is there any pain in your breasts? ___ ___

222. (For women only) Have there been any changes in your nipples? ___ ___

223. (For women only) Have there been any changes in the skin of your breasts? ___ ___

YES NO   YES NO

224. Have you noticed your heart skipping beats or beating rapidly at times in the past few months? — —

247. Do greasy foods upset your stomach? — —

248. Do you have a problem with hemorrhoids? — —

225. Do you get pains in your chest, jaw, shoulders, or down your arms when you climb stairs or hills or walk too fast? — —

249. Do you have to get up more than once a night to urinate? — —

250. Do you have to urinate more than once every three hours during the day? — —

226. Do you ever get such pains at night while lying quietly in bed, or when you get upset? — —

251. Have you had a sense of urgency lately, when having to void, as if you might lose it if you don't rush to the bathroom? — —

227. Have you been getting short of breath lately when you walk more than a block on level ground? — —

252. Do you lose your urine sometimes? — —

253. Have you had a burning sensation lately when you urinate? — —

228. Have you been waking up at night with trouble breathing? — —

254. In the past six months, have you had blood in your urine? — —

229. Do you have to sleep propped up on one or two pillows, or have to sleep sitting up in a chair? — —

255. (For women only) Do you lose your urine sometimes when you laugh, cough, or sneeze? — —

230. Have you had any "blackouts" or "passing out" or "fainting" spells in the past year? — —

256. (For women only) Have you had an itch in your genital area lately? — —

231. Have you had difficulty swallowing or pain when swallowing for more than a month? — —

257. (For women only) Have your periods been much heavier than usual lately (if you still have periods)? — —

232. Have you been nauseated lately? — —

258. (For women only) Have you had any spotting or bleeding between periods lately (if you still have periods)? — —

233. Have you been vomiting lately? — —

234. Have you had black (not just dark), tarry stools in the past six months? — —

259. (For women only) Do you suffer from painful periods (if you still have periods)? — —

235. Have you had pain in the upper abdomen two or more times a week during the past month? — —

260. (For women only) Do you suffer from nervousness or discomfort right before your period begins (if you still have periods)? — —

236. Do you tend to have problems with constipation? — —

261. (For women only) Have you stopped having periods? — —

237. Do your stools tend to be too soft? — —

262. (For women only) Have your periods begun to get lighter or come less often (if you still have periods)? — —

238. Do you tend to have problems with diarrhea? — —

239. Have there been any changes in your bowel habits that have now lasted more than a month? — —

263. (For women only) Do you suffer from "hot flashes" in your face and skin sometimes? — —

240. Have your bowel movements become progressively narrower in size during the past six months? — —

264. (For women only) Do you have vaginal bleeding or spotting? — —

241. Have you noticed any bleeding from the rectum with bowel movements or at other times during the past month? — —

265. (For women only) Have you noticed a foul-smelling discharge lately from your genital area? — —

242. Have you had mucus in your stool with every bowel movement during the past month? — —

266. (For women only) Do you have pain during intercourse? — —

243. Is belching a problem for you? — —

267. Have you noticed that you have lost height since you were younger? — —

244. Does your stomach feel "bloated" often? — —

268. Do you get neck stiffness sometimes? — —

245. Do you tend to pass a lot of gas? — —

246. Do spicy foods upset your stomach? — —

YES NO

269. Do you get pains in the back of your neck sometimes? __ __

270. Do you get lower back pain sometimes? __ __

271. Do you get pains in any other part of your back at times? __ __

272. Do you get pains in your legs when you walk too far? __ __

273. Do your hands turn red, purple, or white sometimes when the weather is cold? __ __

274. Do your feet or ankles swell up sometimes? __ __

275. Do you sometimes suffer from stiffness in any of your joints? __ __

276. Do you sometimes get pains in your hands? __ __

277. Do you sometimes get pains in your elbows? __ __

278. Do you sometimes get pains in your shoulders? __ __

279. Do you sometimes get pains in your hips? __ __

280. Do you sometimes get pains in your knees? __ __

281. Do you sometimes get pains in your ankles? __ __

282. Do you sometimes get pains in your feet? __ __

283. Do you get cramps in your legs at night, or at other times? __ __

284. Do you seem to suffer from forgetfulness? __ __

285. Do you often feel that your mind is not as clear as it used to be? __ __

286. Do you feel that you are a nervous person? __ __

YES NO

287. Do you worry a lot? __ __

288. Do you frequently have trouble sleeping, or think you don't get enough sleep? __ __

289. Do you suffer from nightmares? __ __

290. Have you been feeling depressed lately? __ __

291. Do you feel useless and not needed? __ __

292. Do you often feel lonely even in the presence of others? __ __

293. Do you think others would be better off if you were dead? __ __

294. Do you often feel like crying? __ __

295. Have you noticed any shaking or tremors of your hands or head lately? __ __

296. Have you noticed any tingling in your fingers or toes lately? __ __

297. Have you ever had any weakness of one hand or leg, or of one side of your face, or problems with your ability to talk? __ __

298. Have you ever had any problems with your balance or coordination? __ __

299. Have you ever had any problems with numbness of your face, hands, or feet? __ __

300. Does hot weather bother you more than it does other people? __ __

301. Does cold weather bother you more than it does other people? __ __

302. Do you seem to sweat much more than other people? __ __

303. Do you lose control of your bowels sometimes? __ __

304. Do you have any other health problems? __ __

With the above "yes/no" questions answered, the doctor merely has to know a few descriptive facts to have a fairly thorough medical history. These include such things as your birthplace, education, occupation, retirement age, and family tree details (any diseases your relatives may have had, and the ages at which they died).

The above information does not provide a "complete" medical history in the technical sense of the word. There are many areas which remain uncovered. It is impossible to cover absolutely everything. The questionnaire is an attempt to provide a practical selection of questions which are of the greatest concern to the doctor—particularly the doctor who treats senior citizens.

Appendix B

DOCTOR'S HEALTH SURVEY QUESTIONNAIRE

This second format of the Health Survey Questionnaire is for the benefit of doctors who wish to keep a shorter and more usable form of the Health Survey Questionnaire in their patients' charts. The doctor's version uses medical terminology and abbreviations to which doctors are accustomed. It saves the doctor's time by focusing attention (through bold lettering and thick-lined boxes) on those answers that are of greatest significance. For the most part, the "yes" answers will be of most interest to the doctor. However, a few questions will interest the doctor equally or more if they are answered in the negative. In such instances, the spaces for such negative answers are *also* given thick-lined boxes.

The doctor's version of the questionnaire also includes spaces for a few "open-ended questions" which are important to complete the doctor's history-taking.

DOCTOR'S COMPREHENSIVE INITIAL HISTORY

NAME OF PATIENT _____ DATE _____

	YES NO			YES NO
1. Drug Allergies: _____	☐ —	7. Cholecystectomy		☐ —
2. Other drug reactions: _____	☐ —	8. Appendectomy		☐ —
SURGERY		9. Hernioplasty		☐ —
3. Tonsillectomy	☐ —	10. ICCE		☐ —
4. Hysterectomy	☐ —	11. Other eye surgery		☐ —
5. Marshall-Marchetti	☐ —	12. Skin lesions removed		☐ —
6. Tubal ligation	☐ —	13. Other surgery		☐ —

YES NO

INJURIES

14. Significant head trauma
15. Fractures in general
16. Sprains, whiplash, or other injuries

CHILDHOOD MEDICAL HISTORY

17. Mumps
18. Measles
19. Rubella
20. Chicken pox
21. Other childhood ills
22. Incomplete childhood immunizations
23. Radiation treatment

ADULT MEDICAL HISTORY

24. **Tetanus booster within past 10 years**
25. **Diphtheria booster within past 10 years**
26. **Previous flu shot**
27. **Pneumovax ever given**
28. TB skin test
29. H/o rheumatic fever
30. H/o murmur
31. H/o HTN
32. H/o pneumonia
33. H/o MI
34. H/o GC
35. H/o lues
36. salpingitis
37. genital herpes
38. venereal warts
39. other STDs
40. H/o hepatitis
41. H/o transfusion
42. **Gravida > 0**
43. H/o Ab
44. H/o having breastfed an infant
45. **Recent lab (past few years)**
46. **Recent physical (past few years)**
47. **Pap smear within past few years**
48. H/o abn Pap
49. **Sigmoidoscopy/proctoscopy/colonoscopy hx**
50. H/o biopsy
51. **Previous CXR**

YES NO

52. **Previous EKG**
53. **Monthly BSE not done**
54. **Mammogram within past year**
55. **H/o previous mammogram**
56. H/o B.E.
57. H/o upper GI series
58. H/o oral cholecystogram
59. H/o IVP
60. H/o CT scan or US
61. H/o radiation tx
62. H/o thyroid ca
63. H/o ca larynx
64. H/o oropharyngeal ca
65. H/o emphysema
66. H/o lung ca
67. H/o renal ca
68. H/o bladder ca
69. H/o stomach polyps
70. H/o pernicious anemia
71. H/o ca stomach
72. H/o colorectal polyp
73. H/o ulcerative colitis
74. H/o colon cancer
75. H/o skin cancer
76. **H/o intercourse (female)**
77. H/o mother using DES during pregnancy
78. H/o ca cx
79. H/o endometrial ca
80. H/o ca vagina
81. H/o breast ca
82. H/o having ever been hospitalized

Usual wgt.: _____#.
Maximum wgt. > age 40: _____#.
Minimum wgt. > age 40: _____#.
Maximum height as an adult: _____ ft. _____ in.

SOCIAL HISTORY

Place of Birth: _____

Education: to: _____ (School grade or year of college or grad. education)

Occupation: _____

Date of retirement (if retired): _____

Travel outside the U.S.: _____

83. **Ever married**

If married: separated _____divorced _____
widowed/widower _____

YES NO

84. Live alone

85. Prepare own meals

86. Eat fried foods regularly

87. Eat > 1 egg/wk

88. Eat pork regularly

89. High salt diet

90. Eat bran cereal regularly

91. Smoker

92. Previous smoker

If a smoker, age started _____, age quit _____ / ___
years ago; avg. # ppd. cigarettes smoked: _____
previously, _____ currently; # pack-years _____ .
H/o use of cigars _____, pipe _____,
chewing tobacco _____ .

93. EtOH currently

94. Past h/o EtOH

If a drinker, age started _____, age quit _____ /
_____ years ago; avg. × per week of: _____

	Currently	Previously
4. oz wine	_____	_____
1. oz whiskey	_____	_____
4. oz beer	_____	_____

95. Difficulty shopping for food

96. Financial difficulty affording proper diet

97. Needs assistance with financial affairs

98. Interested relative available for support

99. Interested friend available for support

100. Has Medicare

101. CPR desired if terminal

102. Intubation desired if terminal

103. Tube feeding desired if terminal

104. IV fluids desired if terminal

105. Parental antibiotics desired if terminal

106. Hospitalization desired if terminal

107. CPR desired if severely demented

108. Intubation desired if severely demented

109. Tube feeding desired if severely demented

110. IV fluids desired if severely demented

111. Parental antibiotics desired if severely demented

YES NO

112. Hospitalization desired if severely demented

MEDICATIONS

113. Aspirin used regularly

114. Antacid used

115. Pill for dyspepsia used

116. OTC pain pill used

117. Sleeping pill used

118. "Allergy pill" used

119. "Sinus pill" used

120. "Asthma pill" ever used

121. Hand nembulizer ever used

122. HTN pill ever used

123. K^+ supplement ever used

124. K^+-rich foods deliberately eaten

125. Cardiotonic med taken

126. Diuretic ever used

127. "Thyroid pill" ever used

128. S. L. NTG ever used

129. Topical nitrates ever used

130. Other topical time-released ung. ever used

131. Vasodilator ever used

132. Oral diabetic agents ever used

133. Insulin ever used

134. Rx for seizures ever used

135. Birth control pills ever used

136. Hormones ever used for menopausal sxs

137. Hormones ever used for osteoporosis prevention

138. "Nerve pills" ever used

139. Sleeping pills ever used

140. Diet pills ever used

141. IUD ever used

142. Cream or ung. ever used

143. Vaginal preparation used recently

144. Rectal preparation used recently

145. Vitamins used

146. Iron pills or vitamins with iron used

147. Calcium supplements used

148. Laxatives used

149. Enemas used

150. Stool softeners used

YES NO

151. Eye or ear drops used daily ☐ __

152. Prn eye or ear drops used ☐ __

List of current medications used daily (with strength and directions):

_____

_____

_____

_____

_____

_____

_____

_____

_____

_____

_____

_____

_____

List of current medications used as needed (with strength and directions):

_____

_____

_____

_____

_____

_____

_____

_____

_____

_____

_____

List of previous medications used (with strength and directions):

_____

_____

_____

_____

YES NO

_____

_____

_____

_____

_____

_____

_____

FAMILY HISTORY

153. FH diabetes mellitus ☐ __

154. FH PVD with amputation ☐ __

155. FH HTN ☐ __

156. FH MI ☐ __

157. FH congenital heart disease ☐ __

158. FH heart murmur ☐ __

159. FH angina pectoris ☐ __

160. FH CVA ☐ __

161. FH breast ca ☐ __

162. FH stomach ca ☐ __

163. FH colon polyps ☐ __

164. FH colorectal ca ☐ __

165. FH endometrial ca ☐ __

166. Other FH ca ☐ __

167. FH thyroid problems ☐ __

168. FH urinary tract stones ☐ __

169. FH cholelithiasis ☐ __

170. FH TB ☐ __

171. FH glaucoma ☐ __

172. FH asthma, hay fever, allergies, PCN allergy ☐ __

173. Other FH of note ☐ __

174. FH of suicide ☐ __

Ages at which died:

Mother died of _____

Father died of _____

Siblings are all alive and well ☐

Children are all alive and well ☐

Spouse died in 19__ of _____

Spouse is alive and well ☐

YES NO

REVIEW OF SYSTEMS

General

175. Not independently ambulatory ☐ —
176. Fear of falling ☐ —
177. H/o fall in the past year ☐ —
178. Dizziness ☐ —
179. Fatigue ☐ —
180. Postural dizziness ☐ —
181. Unexplained wt loss > 10 lb/past 6 months ☐ —
182. Declining appetite ☐ —
183. Breast or other lump ☐ —

Skin

184. Bleeding or change in a mole the past 6 mos ☐ —
185. Bleeding or change in a wart the past 6 mos ☐ —
186. Unhealed sore > 1 month's duration ☐ —
187. Skin change in an area of radiation therapy ☐ —
188. Severe burn scar from a burn > a year ago ☐ —
189. Mole in location where it may be irritated ☐ —
190. Fair skin and/or sunburn easily ☐ —
191. Rash ☐ —
192. Itching "all over" lately ☐ —
193. Perineal or rectal itching lately ☐ —

Head

194. Frequent headaches ☐ —
195. Occasional sinusitis headaches ☐ —

Eyes

Last exam by an ophthalmologist: _____ mos / years ago

196. Glasses used ☐ —
197. Contact lenses used ☐ —
198. Itchy eyes ☐ —
199. Watery eyes ☐ —
200. Reduced vision ☐ —

Ears

201. Reduced hearing ☐ —
202. Audiometry ever done ☐ —
203. Stuffy ears ☐ —
204. Itchy ears ☐ —

YES NO

205. Otic discharge ☐ —
206. Tinnitus ☐ —

Nose

207. Frequent rhinorrhea or stuffy nose ☐ —
208. Frequent epistaxis ☐ —

Mouth and Throat

Last dental visit: _____ mos / years ago

209. Dental caries ☐
210. Oral cavity irritation from dentures or teeth ☐
211. Oral pain or tenderness present > 1 mo ☐
212. Possible leukoplakia present > 1 mo ☐
213. Voice change/hoarseness present > 1 mo ☐

Neck

214. Pressure in thyroid area > 1 mo ☐

Chest

215. Daily cough > 1 mo ☐ —
216. Hemoptysis within the past month ☐ —
217. Frequent chest congestion ☐ —
218. Wheezing ☐ —
219. Productive cough ☐ —
220. Other breathing problems ☐ —

(For Women Only) Breasts

221. Breast pain currently ☐ —
222. Nipple changes ☐ —
223. Skin changes of the breasts ☐ —

Heart

224. Irregular or rapid heartbeat ☐ —
225. Exertional angina ☐ —
226. Angina at night or with anxiety ☐ —
227. DOE 1 block level ground ☐ —
228. PND ☐ —
229. Orthopnea ☐ —
230. Syncope in the past year ☐ —

Digestive

231. Dysphagia present > 1 mo ☐ —
232. Nausea ☐ —
233. Vomiting ☐ —
234. Melena within past 6 mos ☐ —
235. Epigastric pain ≥ twice a week during past month ☐

YES NO

236. Constipation ☐ —
237. Stools too soft ☐ —
238. Diarrhea ☐ —
239. Change in bowel habits present more than a month ☐ —

On the average, bowels move _____×/day; every ___ days

240. Narrowing of stool during past 6 months ☐ —
241. BRBPPR within past month ☐ —
242. Mucus in all stools the past month ☐ —
243. Belching ☐ —
244. Bloated feeling ☐ —
245. Flatulence ☐ —
246. Intol. to spicy foods ☐ —
247. Intol. to greasy foods ☐ —
248. Hemorrhoids ☐ —

Genitourinary

249. Nocturia ☐ —
250. Frequency ☐ —
251. Urgency ☐ —
252. Urinary incontinence ☐ —
253. Dysuria ☐ —
254. Gross hematuria within the past 6 mos ☐ —
255. Stress incontinence ☐ —
256. Vaginal itch ☐ —
257. Menorrhagia ☐ —
258. Metrorrhagia ☐ —
259. Dysmenorrhea ☐ —
260. Premenstrual syndrome ☐ —
261. Amenorrhea ☐ —
262. Onset of menopause ☐ —
263. Hot flashes ☐ —
264. Unexplained vaginal bleeding ☐ —
265. Purulent vaginal discharge ☐ —
266. Dyspareunia ☐ —

Back and Spine

267. Loss of height ☐ —
268. Neck stiffness ☐ —
269. Neck pains ☐ —

YES NO

270. Low back pains ☐ —
271. Other back pains ☐ —

Extremities

272. Intermittent claudication ☐ —
273. Raynaud's syndrome ☐ —
274. Pedal or ankle edema ☐ —
275. Joint stiffness ☐ —
276. Pains in hands ☐ —
277. Pains in elbows ☐ —
278. Pains in shoulders ☐ —
279. Pains in hips ☐ —
280. Pains in knees ☐ —
281. Pains in ankles ☐ —
282. Pains in feet ☐ —
283. Leg cramps ☐ —

Neuro-Psychiatric

284. Forgetfulness ☐ —
285. Confusion ☐ —
286. Anxiety ☐ —
287. Anxiety ☐ —
288. Sleeping difficulties ☐ —
289. Nightmares ☐ —
290. Depressed ☐ —
291. Depressed ☐ —
292. Depressed ☐ —
293. Depressed ☐ —
294. Depressed ☐ —
295. Head or hand tremors ☐ —
296. Peripheral neuropathy (tingling) ☐ —
297. Focal weakness or dysphasia ☐ —
298. Poor balance or incoordination ☐ —
299. Sensory loss, face or extremities ☐ —

Autonomic

300. Heat intolerance ☐ —
301. Cold intolerance ☐ —
302. Hyperhidrosis ☐ —
303. Fecal incontinence ☐ —
304. Other health problems ☐ —

Appendix C

FOODS HIGH IN CALCIUM

The best sources of foods high in calcium are milk and dairy products, such as ice cream and cheese. The lactose in milk enhances the absorption of calcium. Calcium absorption is also enhanced by vitamin D, with which most milk is fortified.

Here is a list of the calcium content of a number of calcium-rich foods. For recommendations on how much calcium per day is appropriate, see Chapter 9.

Food	Mg of Calcium per Serving
Vanilla milkshake	457
Plain yogurt	415
Chocolate milkshake	396
Flavored low-fat yogurt	389
Sardines with bones	372
Malted milk	347
Fruit yogurt	345
Part skim milk ricotta cheese	337
Cheese pizza	332
Skim milk	302
1% low-fat milk	300
2% low-fat milk	297
Whole milk	291
Buttermilk	285
Chocolate milk	284
Swiss cheese	272
Monterey cheese	212
Edam cheese	207
Swiss cheese (pasteurized)	205
Cheddar cheese	204

Muenster cheese	203
Colby cheese	194
Cream of mushroom soup (made from milk)	191
Caraway cheese	191
Brick cheese	191
Mozarella cheese (part skim milk)	183
Macaroni and cheese	181
Waffle	179
Collard greens, from raw collard	179
Beef taco	174
American cheese (pasteurized)	174
Cream of tomato soup (made from milk)	168
Salmon with bones	167
Cheese food, American (pasteurized)	163
Blue cheese	150
Collards, from frozen	149
Spaghetti with meatballs, tomato sauce, and cheese	148
Tofu, processed with calcium sulfate	145
Molasses, blackstrap	137
Pudding, chocolate	133
Ice milk, soft serve	127
Bokchoy	126
Turnip greens, from raw	125
Pancakes	116
Oysters, raw	113
Kale, from raw	103
Shrimp, canned	99
Turnip greens, from frozen	98
Mustard greens	97
Cornbread	94
Beans, cooked dried	90
Ice milk	88
Ice cream	88
Chili concarne with beans	82
Kale, from frozen	79
Cottage cheese, 2% low fat	77

Appendix D

FOODS HIGH IN SALT

As discussed in various chapters in this book, it is very important for certain individuals to reduce their salt intake, particularly those persons who have high blood pressure, congestive heart failure, or swelling of the lower legs. Additionally, it is generally believed that reducing the amount of salt ingested is a healthy thing for most everyone, simply because most Americans take in—on the average—about 20 times more salt than they need to. The way salt does its damage is by causing the body to retain more fluid than necessary, through a process known as "osmosis." One way of explaining this process is that excessive salt "fools the body" into thinking it is dehydrated, causing it to retain additional water.

It is not just ordinary table salt that can be bad for you. Persons who need to restrict salt need to restrict *sodium in any form*. It is the sodium in table salt which causes all the harm. Some forms of salt—such as potassium salt—contain no sodium at all. Common sources of sodium other than "salt" are monosodium glutamate, baking powder, baking soda, sodium sulfite, sodium nitrate or nitrite, sodium benzoate, and disodium phosphate. The symbol "Na^+"—for "sodium"—is also to be looked out for, as "Na" in any chemical combination causes fluid retention by the body.

Salt is present naturally in most foods, even though they may not taste "salty." It is also added to many foods, either by manufacturers during processing, or by chefs during cooking. And, of course, many people add "table salt" to their food after it is prepared. In fact, about 25 percent of the salt people ingest is what they sprinkle on after the food is prepared.

Because sodium is the real culprit in causing fluid retention, and since sodium comes in combinations other than just sodium chloride, salt content is typically measured in milligrams of *sodium*. Occasionally, however, milligrams of *salt* are mentioned. To calculate the number of milligrams of sodium in table salt, you multiply by .40. Thus, 10,000 mg of table salt contains 4,000 mg of sodium. Another useful fact to remember is that there are 1,000 mg in a gram. Thus, a 2,000-mg-a-day sodium restriction is sometimes referred to as a "2 gram sodium diet."

Precisely how much one should restrict sodium depends on whether there is any medical condition, such as high blood pressure or congestive heart failure. In such case, your doctor should be consulted. Persons with high blood pressure are typically advised to follow a 2,000-mg-per-day sodium limit. Persons with congestive heart failure sometimes must limit themselves to even less sodium—as little as 500 to 1,000 mg a day.

The Food and Nutrition Board of the National Research Council believes the ideal range for most adults is from 1,100 to 3,000 mg a day of sodium. In contrast, Americans typically ingest from 4,000 to 10,000 mg of sodium a day.

A mild restriction is 3 grams (3,000 mg) of sodium per day; 2,000 mg is a moderate restriction, 1,000 mg is a severe restriction, and 500 mg or less is a very severe restriction. Restrictions of 1,000 mg a day and less are difficult to adhere to because food loses much of its palatability at this range. However, the use of herbs and spices can do much to compensate for this loss of flavor.

The following general guidelines will help you to avoid ingesting a large amount of sodium in your diet:

- Add salt to your food cautiously, if at all.
- Minimize the amount of salt you use in your cooking.
- Cut down on processed foods, such as "fast foods," canned foods, "convenience" foods, and packaged foods.
- Be careful of food additives. Read the labels on foods and medicines.

Salt substitutes generally contain potassium and should never be used without first checking with your doctor. Older persons sometimes suffer from some degree of silent kidney failure which could make salt substitutes dangerous to use. You should also be aware that "Lite Salt" is a combination of sodium and potassium salts, and therefore is not free of sodium.

As of July 1986, new Food and Drug Administration regulations allow manufacturers to classify products, based on sodium content, in the following ways:

- **Sodium free:** less than 5 mg of sodium per serving
- **Very low sodium:** 35 mg of sodium or less per serving
- **Low sodium:** 140 mg of sodium or less per serving
- **Reduced sodium:** one-quarter or less the amount of sodium compared to comparable foods

The best way to reduce your sodium intake is to learn which foods are high in sodium, and avoid them. To this end, we here present two listings—a general one and a specific one. You may find each of them helpful.

FOODS OR CATEGORIES OF FOODS HIGH IN SODIUM*

Soups
Bouillon cubes
Canned broth
Dried soup mixes
Instant noodle mixes, such as
  Top Ramen

Vegetables
Canned vegetables
Canned tomato juice
Canned vegetable juice
Frozen peas
Frozen lima beans
Frozen vegetables with
  seasoned sauce
Olives
Pickled vegetables
Pickles
Sauerkraut
Seaweed

High Protein Foods
Bacon
Canned meats

Corned beef
Dried chipped beef
Ham, cured or "low salt"
Hot dogs
Luncheon meats
Salt pork
Sausage
Smoked meats
Salted or pickled meats
Meat extenders and "helpers"
TV and frozen dinners
"Fast food" meats
Anchovies
Canned fish
Commercially frozen fish
"Fast food" fish
Herring
Salted fish
Sardines
Smoked or pickled fish
TV and frozen fish dinners
Crab prepared with salty seasoning
Mussels

* Partially adapted from L. Randol Barker, M.D., John R. Burton, M.D., and Philip D. Zieve, M.D., *Principles of Ambulatory Medicine*, 2nd edition (Baltimore: Williams & Wilkins, 1986), which in turn was adapted from "Health Is In—Salt Is Out," courtesy of the Maryland High Blood Pressure Coordinating Council.

Scallops
Canned chicken
Canned turkey
Commercial fried chicken
TV dinners
Turkey roll
Frozen turkey or chicken casseroles/
  pies
Frozen omelet
Frozen souffle
Frozen quiche

Breads, Crackers, Cereals, Grains
Biscuits
Cornbread
Packaged croutons
Danish pastries
Muffins
Pancakes
Stuffing mix
Sweet rolls
Waffles
Crackers with salted tops
Pretzels
Soda crackers
Instant grits; Instant hot cereals
Certain dry cereals (check the labels)
Chow mein noodles
Prepackaged meals, such as maca-
  roni, noodle, or spaghetti dinners

Fruits
Dried fruits that contain sodium preservatives

Commercially Prepared Desserts
Cakes
Cookies
Donuts
Pie

Pudding mixes
Sweet rolls

Seasonings
Barbecue sauce
Catsup
Celery salt
Chili sauce
Cooking wine (has salt added)
Garlic salt
Lemon pepper seasoning
Meat tenderizers
Monosodium glutamate (MSG)
Onion salt
Pickle relish
Prepared mustard
Seasoned or plain salt
Sea salt
Soy sauce
Steak sauce

Dairy Products
Buttermilk (commercial)
Condensed milk
"Fast food" shakes
Blue cheese
Camembert cheese
Processed cheese, both American
  and Swiss
Processed cheese foods
Processed cheese spreads
Provolone
Roquefort cheese
Parmesan cheese
Feta cheese
Gouda cheese
Edam cheese
Romano cheese
Tilsit cheese

SODIUM CONTENT OF SELECTED FOODS*

Food	Size Portion	Mg Sodium
Smoked herring	3 oz	5,234
Fermented (miso) soybeans, red	¼ cup	3,708
Chicken dinner (fast food)	1 portion	2,243
Fermented (miso) soybeans, white	¼ cup	2,126
Pancake mix	1 cup	2,036
Sweet and sour canned pork	1 cup	1,968
Canned shrimp	3 oz	1,955
Table salt	1 tsp	1,938
Swedish meatballs	8 oz	1,880
Garlic salt	1 tsp	1,850
Veal parmigiana	7.5 oz	1,825
Meat tenderizer	1 tsp	1,750
Onion salt	1 tsp	1,620
Sauerkraut, canned	1 cup	1,554
Corned beef hash, canned	1 cup	1,520
Chicken and dumplings, frozen	12 oz	1,506
Tomato sauce	1 cup	1,498
Canned Spanish rice	1 cup	1,370
Frozen meatloaf dinner	1 dinner	1,304
Chicken noodle soup, dehydrated, with water	1 cup	1,284
Frozen vegetable chow mein without meat	1 cup	1,273
Frozen turkey dinner	1 dinner	1,228
Green pea soup, dehydrated, with water	1 cup	1,220
Dried, chipped beef	3 oz	1,219
Frozen fish dinner	1 dinner	1,212
Cashews, salted dry roasted	1 cup	1,200
Chili concarne with beans, canned	1 cup	1,185
Canned beef and macaroni prepared dish	1 cup	1,185
Frozen chicken dinner	1 dinner	1,153
Vegetable soup, dehydrated, with water	1 cup	1,146
Stuffing mix, cooked	1 cup	1,131
Ham	3 oz	1,114
Chicken noodle soup, condensed, with water	1 cup	1,107
Potatoes, au gratin	1 cup	1,095
Frozen pot pie	1 pie	1,093
Mushroom soup, condensed, with milk	1 cup	1,076
Canned ravioli	7.5 oz	1,065

* The information in this table is adapted from "The Sodium Content of Your Food," Home and Garden Bulletin Number 233 of The United States Department of Agriculture (August 1980).

Canned spaghetti and ground beef	7.5 oz	1,054
Beef noodle soup, dehydrated, with water	1 cup	1,041
Canned Goulash prepared dish	8 oz	1,032
Mushroom soup, condensed, with water	1 cup	1,031
Soy sauce	1 tbsp	1,029
Manhattan clam chowder, condensed, with water	1 cup	1,029
Mushroom soup, dehydrated, with water	1 cup	1,019
Stuffed frozen peppers	8 oz	1,001
Vegetable beef soup, dehydrated, with water	1 cup	1,000
Frozen beef dinner	1 dinner	998
New England clam chowder, condensed, with milk	1 cup	992
Jumbo hamburger (fast food)		990
Green pea soup, condensed, with water	1 cup	987
Peanuts, salted dry roasted	1 cup	986
Chicken rice soup, dehydrated, with water	1 cup	980
Canned stew	8 oz	980
Chopped sirloin frozen dinner	1 dinner	978
Frozen pizza with sausage	½ pie	967
Vegetable beef soup, condensed, with water	1 cup	957
Beef noodle soup, condensed, with water	1 cup	952
Tomato soup, dehydrated, with water	1 cup	943
Canned spaghetti and meatballs	7.5 oz	942
Tomato soup, condensed, with milk	1 cup	932
Dill pickles	1 pickle	928
New England clam chowder, condensed, with water	1 cup	914
Beans, Italian, canned	1 cup	913
Minestrone soup, condensed, with water	1 cup	911
Spinach, canned	1 cup	910
Canned corned beef	3 oz	893
Vegetable juice cocktail	1 cup	887
Fish sandwich (fast food)		882
Tomato juice	1 cup	878
Tomato soup, condensed, with water	1 cup	872
Canned spaghetti sauce	4 oz	856
Vegetable soup, condensed, with water	1 cup	823
Peanuts, salted Spanish	1 cup	823
Baking soda	1 tsp	821
Chicken rice soup, condensed, with water	1 cup	814
Frozen pizza with pepperoni	½ pie	813
Cooked corned beef	3 oz	802
Summer squash, canned	1 cup	785
Frozen shrimp dinner	1 dinner	758
Potatoes, canned	1 cup	753

Food	Size Portion	Mg. Sodium
Enchiladas, prepared dish	1 pkg	725
Chow mein, home recipe	1 cup	718
Tuna pot pie	1 pie	715
Canned roasted chicken products	5 oz can	714
Cheeseburger (fast food)		709
Teriyaki sauce	1 tbsp	690
Knockwurst	1 link	687
Swiss steak frozen dinner	1 dinner	682
Macaroni salad	⅔ cup	676
Frozen beef and macaroni prepared dish	6 oz	673
Corn, cream style, canned	1 cup	671
Frozen chicken and noodles	¾ cup	662
Frozen egg roll	1 roll	648
Home baked pot pie	1 pie	644
Meat frankfurter	1	639
Potatoes, mashed, with milk and salt	1 cup	632
Potato salad	½ cup	625
Home recipe pot pie	1 pie	620
Chicken frankfurter	1	617
Peanuts, salted, roasted	1 cup	601
Tomatos, stewed, canned	1 cup	584
Corn, vacuum pack, canned	1 cup	577
Canned drained sardines	3 oz	552
Bean salad, canned	½ cup	537
Grated parmesan cheese	1 oz	528
Roquefort cheese	1 oz	513
Carrots, frozen, with brown sugar glaze	3.3 oz	500
Peas, green, canned	1 cup	493
MSG (monosodium glutamate)	1 tsp	492
Potatoes, instant, reconstituted	1 cup	485
Sliced beets, canned	1 cup	479
Instant, whole milk chocolate pudding	½ cup	470
Hamburger (fast food)		461
Regular and low-fat cottage cheese	4 oz	457
Beans, lima, canned	1 cup	456
Hard parmesan cheese	1 oz	454
Cheese pizza	¼ 12-inch pie	447
Instant whole butterscotch pudding	½ cup	445
Pink canned salmon, salt added	3 oz	443
Broccoli, frozen, with cheese sauce	1 cup	440
Canned bonito fish	3 oz	437
Canned, drained crab	3 oz	425
Brussels sprouts, frozen, in butter sauce	3.3 oz	421

Peas, green, frozen, in cream sauce	2.6 oz	420
American cheese	1 oz	406
Peas, green, frozen, in butter sauce	3.3 oz	402
Devil's food cake, from mix	¹⁄₁₂ cake	402
Taco (fast food)		401
Instant, whole-milk vanilla pudding	½ cup	400
Raw salt pork	1 oz	399
Cubed beef broth	1 cup	396
Blue cheese	1 oz	396
Canadian bacon	1 slice	394
Tomatoes, whole, canned	1 cup	390
Sweetened, condensed, evaporated canned milk	1 cup	389
Swiss cheese	1 oz	388
Solid oil-pack white meat canned tuna	3 oz	384
Corn, whole-kernel canned	1 cup	384
Ham and cheese loaf	1 oz	381
Mixed vegetables, canned	1 cup	380
Beans, snap, with onions	3 oz	360
Total cereal	1 cup	359
Wheaties cereal	1 cup	355
Instant hominy grits cooked in unsalted water	¾ cup	354
Mix'n eat cream of wheat cereal	¾ cup	350
Carrots, frozen, in butter sauce	3.3 oz	350
Dough roll, refrigerated		342
Rice Krispies	1 cup	340
Baking powder	1 tsp	339
Canned sardines in tomato sauce	3 oz	338
Beans, snap, with almonds	3 oz	335
Pickled beets, canned	1 cup	330
Canned red salmon, salt added	3 oz	329
Frosted cinnamon toaster pastry		326
Beans, snap, canned	1 cup	326
Cauliflower, frozen, with cheese sauce	3 oz	325
Frosted apple toaster pastry		324
Olives, green	4 olives	323
Frozen oysters	3 oz	323
Regular nonfat dry milk	½ cup	322
Feta cheese	1 oz	316
Bratwurst	1 oz	315
Steamed crab	3 oz	314
Olive loaf (luncheon meat spread)	1 slice	312
Buttermilk	½ cup	310
Water pack solid white meat canned tuna	3 oz	309
Raisin Bran cereal	½ cup	304

Food	*Size Portion*	*Mg. Sodium*
Oil pack light meat, chunk canned tuna	3 oz	303
Silver canned salmon, salt added	3 oz	298
Asparagus, canned	4 spears	298
Corn Chex cereal	1 cup	297
Skim evaporated milk	1 cup	294
English muffin	1 medium	293
Ready-to-serve butterscotch pudding	½ cup	290
Water pack light meat, chunk canned tuna	3 oz	288
Chopped ham	1 slice	288
Instant oatmeal, sodium added	¾ cup	283
Spinach, frozen creamed	3 oz	280
Ready-to-serve vanilla pudding	1 can	279
Instant oatmeal with maple and brown sugar	¾ cup	277
Harvard beets, canned	1 cup	275
A-1 sauce	1 tbsp	275
Sugar-coated corn flakes	¾ cup	274
Cooked bacon	2 slices	274
Baking powder biscuits with milk from mix	1 biscuit	272
Potatoes, frozen, salted	2.5 oz	270
Whole evaporated canned milk	1 cup	266
Milkshake (fast food)		266
Special K cereal	1-¼ cup	265
Smoked sausage	1 link	264
Ready-to-serve chocolate pudding	1 can	262
Bran Chex cereal	⅔ cup	262
Frozen cinnamon Danish pastry	1 roll	260
One-step angel food cake, from mix	1/12 cake	259
Mince pie, frozen	⅛ of pie	258
Ham spread	1 oz	258
Salted buttermilk	1 cup	257
Regular Cornflakes cereal	1 cup	256
Cooked beef salami	1 slice	255
Dry mix, prepared French dressing	1 tbsp	253
Deviled ham	1 oz	253
40% Bran cereal	⅔ cup	251
Frozen cheese Danish	1 roll	250
Provolone cheese	1 oz	248
Grated canned tuna	3 oz	246
Regular whole milk butterscotch pudding	½ cup	245
Raw mussels	3 oz	243
Yellow cake from mix	1/12 cake	242
Mushrooms, canned	2 oz	242
Frosted blueberry toaster pastry		242

Pecan pie, frozen	⅛ of pie	241
Peas, green, frozen, with mushrooms	3.3 oz	240
Camembert cheese	1 oz	239
White cake from mix	1/12 cake	238
Strawberry toaster pastry		238
Rice Chex cereal	1-⅛ cup	238
Cooked beef and pork salami	1 slice	234
Cocoa mix, water added	8 fl oz	232
Summer squash, frozen, with curry	⅓ cup	228
Roasted duck (flesh and skin)	½ duck	227
Chili	1 tbsp	227
Pork salami, dry or hard	1 slice	226
Steamed scallops	3 oz	225
Beef and pork bologna	1 slice	224
Instant oatmeal with raisins and spice	¾ cup	223
100% bran cereal	½ cup	221
Instant oatmeal with apples and cinnamon	¾ cup	220
Frozen apple Danish	1 roll	220
Beef bologna	1 slice	220
Raw scallops	3 oz	217
Pork and beef cooked sausage	1 patty	217
Natural flavor malted milk	1 cup	215
Bottled French dressing	1 tbsp	214
Boiled lobster	3 oz	212
Dried, sulfured apples	8 oz	210
Baked custard	1 cup	209
Apple pie, frozen	⅛ of pie	208
Worcestershire sauce	1 tbsp	206
Flounder, sole, flat fish baked w/butter	3 oz	201
Regular, whole-milk vanilla pudding	½ cup	200

SODIUM CONTENT OF SELECTED DRUGS

Product	Mg Sodium
Sal Hepatica	1,000
Bromo-Seltzer	717
Alka-Seltzer (blue box)	521
Alka-Seltzer (gold box)	276
Fleet's Enema	275

Appendix E

FOODS HIGH IN POTASSIUM

The most common circumstances for needing to increase one's intake of potassium-rich foods are the following:

- Being placed on "water pills," which drain potassium from the body. Such pills are commonly prescribed for persons with high blood pressure, congestive heart failure, or swelling of the lower legs. Increasing one's potassium intake is particularly important for such persons who also have certain other medical conditions like diabetes or angina pectoris, or who are also taking digitalis preparations.

- Being a "potassium-waster." Some people just "naturally" tend to lose an excessive amount of potassium through the kidneys. In many cases this is the result of many years of heavy drinking—even though they may no longer be drinking currently. A blood test shows that the person's potassium level is low.

- Laxative abuse, or a bout of diarrhea. Considerable quantities of potassium can be lost through the stool in persons who suffer from several days of diarrhea, or who abuse certain laxatives on a daily basis.

A classic sign of being low in potassium is leg cramps. However, not all persons with leg cramps have them because of being low in potassium. Persons with poor arterial circulation to the legs tend to get leg cramps, particularly at night. Increasing one's potassium intake will not relieve that problem. Other signs of low potassium are cramps in the hands or forearms, generalized weakness, feeling lethargic or "run down," a "tired feeling" in the front of the thighs, mental confusion, depression, and erratic beating of the heart.

No older person should make radical changes in diet—especially with respect to increasing the amounts of potassium-rich foods—without being under a doctor's supervision. Before one begins to eat a diet high in potassium-rich foods, it is important to be sure that one's kidneys are able to clear out "waste products," including *excess potassium,* adequately. Very old persons especially may suffer from some degree of kidney failure, and can easily accumulate *too much* potassium in their bloodstream. It can be dangerous for such persons to eat too many potassium-rich foods or take potassium supplements. Unlike the condition of low potassium, the condition of too high potassium in the blood has few if any warning signs. The first clue that something is seriously wrong may be a dangerous fluttering of the heart muscle.

In contrast with sodium intake (discussed in Appendix D), the average person's dietary intake of potassium—about 2,500 to 4,000 mg per day—is just about what is needed for normal functioning. However, when persons are placed on "water pills," they typically lose about 500 to 1,000 mg per day of potassium through the urine. For people whose diet is already low in potassium, increasing the intake of foods high in potassium may be important.

It is important to have a clear understanding of the underlying purpose for increasing one's potassium intake before deciding to eat more foods high in potassium. In most cases, persons who need more potassium are taking diuretics (water pills) to remove sodium (and with it, through osmotic effect, water) from the body. Eating certain potassium-rich foods that are also very high in *sodium*—such as canned tomato juice or most canned vegetables—will negate the effects of the water pill. Therefore, it is usually important to know not just the *potassium* content of potassium-rich foods, but their *sodium* content, as well. For this reason, the following potassium-rich foods are divided into two lists: those with negligible sodium content and those with significant sodium content.

POTASSIUM-RICH FOODS
WITH NEGLIGIBLE SODIUM CONTENT*

Food	Portion Size	Potassium Content (in mg)
Prunes, dried	10 medium	694
Dates	10 pitted	647
Avocado	½ pitted	604
Watermelon	1 slice	601
Prune juice	1 cup	585
Orange juice	**1 cup**	**484**
Winter squash	½ cup boiled	464
Lima beans	⅝ cup	421
Cooked dried beans	½ cup	417
Grapefruit juice	1 cup	406
Banana	**1**	**370**
Tomato (fresh)	1 medium	367
Pineapple juice	1 cup	359
Potato, sweet	1 boiled	300
Plum	2 medium	300
Orange	1 small	300
Potato, white	1 boiled	285
Apricots	3 medium	281
Brussels sprouts	7 medium	273
Pear	1 medium	261
Honeydew melon	¼ small	250
Cantaloupe	¼ medium	250
Peach	1 medium	203
Corn	1 ear	195
Fruit cocktail	½ cup	168
Strawberries	10 large	164
Grapefruit	½ medium	137
Peanuts, roasted	1 tablespoon	117
Apple	1 medium	109
Raisins	1 tablespoon	78
Peanut butter	2 tablespoons	78
Mixed nuts	3½ oz	78
Applesauce	⅓ cup	66

* Adapted from Table 45.2, "Some Common Potassium-Rich Foods," in L. Randol Barker, M.D., John R. Burton, M.D., and Philip D. Zieve, M.D., *Principles of Ambulatory Medicine*, 2nd edition (Baltimore: Williams & Wilkins, 1986).

Note: Items commonly referred to by doctors when discussing foods in these categories are emphasized with bold-faced type.

POTASSIUM-RICH FOODS
WITH SIGNIFICANT SODIUM CONTENT*

Food	Portion Size	Potassium Content (in mg)	Sodium Content (in mg)
Artichoke	1 large	858	51
Vegetable juice	1 cup	550	304
Tomato juice	**1 cup**	**534**	**293**
Rib roast	2 slices	437	24
Hamburger	1 patty	382	24
Whole milk	8 oz	351	70
Skim milk	8 oz	332	84
Buttermilk	8 oz	312	196
Fish	1 medium filet	312	108
Clams	4 large	234	24
Tomato, canned	½ cup	218	46
Oysters	6 medium	121	43

Note: Items commonly referred to by doctors when discussing foods in these categories are emphasized with bold-faced type.

As you can see from the above tables, tomato juice is not such a good source of potassium for people taking "water pills" because of its relatively high sodium content. On the other hand, such common foods as orange juice and bananas are excellent sources of potassium for such persons. A glass or two per day of orange juice will replenish the lost potassium from mild diuretics, for most persons.

One should be aware that there is a limit to how much potassium one can push in one's diet, when it comes to replacing the potassium which "water pills" cause the body to lose. This is not strictly a matter of quantity. It is because the potassium in foods is mostly in the form of potassium *phosphate* or potassium *citrate*, whereas the potassium which is lost by the body because of water pills is in the form of potassium *chloride*. Therefore, to be fully effective, potassium replacements must likewise be in the form of potassium *chloride*. Because of this, it is necessary for doctors to prescribe potassium supplements, in the form of potassium chloride, for patients who must take large doses of "water pills." Simply modifying the diet will not suffice.

Appendix F

FOODS HIGH IN PURINES

Gout, a condition discussed in Chapter 10, tends to become a problem for many older persons whose kidneys begin to fail. The reason is that the kidneys can no longer clear uric acid from the bloodstream as quickly as necessary. An excess buildup of uric acid in the blood can result in an attack of gout. Persons who tend to get gout should follow a diet low in purines—the chemical compound that breaks down into uric acid in the body.

Another group of persons who tend to get gout are those who already have an underlying tendency (either from heredity or kidney failure, or both) and who change their diet to include more high-fiber foods. Since certain high-fiber foods are also high in purines, such persons are sometimes surprised to find themselves afflicted with this malady for the first time. They may need to become versed in which high-fiber foods are also high in purines, and avoid them.

The following foods are extremely high in purines:

Sardines	Heart
Anchovies	Tongue
Mackerel	Brains
Herring	Sweetbreads
Scallops	Goose
Mussels	Wild game
Partridge	Meat broth
Roe (caviar)	Meat drippings
Liver	Gravy
Kidney	Yeast

The following foods are moderately high in purines:

Shellfish (other than mussels)	Lentils
Eels	Dried beans (including
Other fish	lima beans)
Poultry	Dried peas
Meat	Spinach
Meat soups	Oatmeal
Asparagus	Wheat germ and bran

The following foods have only a modestly elevated purine content:

All fruits	Milk
Vegetables, except those listed above	Milk and fruit desserts
Most breads and cereals	Cheese
All nuts	Eggs
All kinds of fats	Sugars, syrups, sweets
Gelatin	Vegetable and cream soups

Persons with a tendency to gout should also follow certain other dietary guidelines which help prevent the buildup of uric acid in the body.

- Avoid becoming dehydrated. This means drinking plenty of fluids—at least eight cups of liquid per day—and limiting alcohol, caffeine, and tea, which tend to cause increased urination.

- Limit the use of fats and oils, which tend to interfere with the elimination of uric acid from the body. This means avoiding fried foods, fatty meats, gravies and cream sauces, cream, chocolate, ice cream, nuts, and other high-fat snacks.

- Avoid fasting, because this causes the body to break down its own protein into uric acid.

- Gradually reduce to achieve ideal body weight if overweight, since obesity tends to increase uric acid levels.

- Limit daily protein intake to 1 gram per kilogram of ideal body weight. This would be about 70 to 80 grams per day.

Appendix G

FOODS HIGH IN IRON

The greatest problem with iron is that some people think it can cure everything. If they do not have enough energy, they become convinced it is because of "tired blood," which is deficient in iron. As a result, they begin to take iron supplements without a doctor's recommendation. In fact, iron deficiency in healthy persons who eat a balanced diet is unusual. When there is a deficiency of iron, it is usually a sign of something which needs medical investigation. Colon cancer is one common cause in older persons (see Chapter 3). Another is stomach or duodenal ulcers (see Chapter 17). Persons who do suffer from anemia due to iron deficiency must have the cause investigated. If the cause is colon cancer, the cure is to remove the cancer; taking iron pills will not stop internal bleeding from the tumor. If a doctor does find evidence of internal bleeding (blood in the stool) and a thorough investigation finds it is due to something relatively innocuous, such as diverticulosis ("potholes" in the intestine, which tend to bleed from time to time), then it may well be necessary for such persons to take iron supplements or increase the amount of iron in their diet. Because excessive amounts of iron over a long period of time can lead to scarring of the liver, any increase in your iron intake should be recommended by your doctor.

Only about 5 to 10 percent of the iron in food is actually absorbed. The iron in "animal products" (such as meat, poultry, and fish) is absorbed the best—about 25 to 35 percent. The iron in eggs, grains, fruits and vegetables is absorbed much more poorly— only about 2 to 20 percent. Vitamin C—either as a supplement or via foods—enhances the absorption of iron. Factors present in meat also increase iron absorption. If iron-rich foods other than meat are eaten at the same time, such factors will increase the amount of iron absorbed from the other foods.

The recommended dietary allowance (RDA) of iron for males over 18 and for women over 50 is 10 mg per day. The RDA is somewhat higher—18 mg per day—for females from age 11 to 50.

The following is a list of the iron content in various foods.*

Food	Portion Size	Iron Content (in mg)
Total, or Product 19 cereal	1 oz	17–18
Cream of Wheat cereal	¾ cup	7.7
Beef liver, cooked	3 oz	7.5
Life, 40% Bran Flakes, Kix cereal	1 oz	7–8
Oatmeal, Instant, Fortified	1 pkt. (6 oz)	6.3
Clams, raw	3 oz	5.2
Oysters, raw	3 oz (6 medium)	4.8
Wheat Chex, Cheerios, Raisin Bran, Special K cereal	1 oz.	4–6
Apricots, dried	½ cup	3.8
Spinach, cooked	½ cup	3.2
Roast beef, cooked	3 oz	3.1
Potato, baked	1 medium	2.8
Hamburger, cooked	3 oz pattie	2.6
Sardines, canned	3 oz	2.5
Soybeans, cooked	½ cup	2.3
Lima beans, cooked	½ cup	2.1
Almonds	½ cup chopped	1.9
Raisins	½ cup	1.7
Tuna, canned	3 oz	1.6
Prune juice	½ cup	1.5
Spaghetti, enriched, cooked	1 cup	1.4
Peas, cooked	½ cup	1.2
Peanut butter	4 tbsp.	1.2
Ham	3 oz	1.2
Squash, acorn, cooked	½ cup	1.0
Egg	1 large	1.0
Chicken, cooked	3 oz	1.0
Brussels sprouts, cooked	½ cup	1.0
Dandelion greens, cooked	½ cup	0.9
Broccoli, cooked	½ cup	0.9
Tomato juice	½ cup	0.7
Bread, enriched or whole wheat	1 slice	0.7

* Adapted from *Iron, It's in Your Blood,* Safeway's Nutrition Awareness Program.

INDEX

341

DATE DUE